FORWARD

This is the beginning of the end.

It is the end of 40 years of gross human rights abuse against persons living with Lyme and relapsing fever borreliosis and other coinfections from tick borne diseases.

It is the end of State actors promoting policies that:
- obstruct access to treatment options that meet internationally accepted standards;
- obstruct access to antimicrobials for systemic infections in the brain and nervous system;
- encourage the misapplication of fraudulent psychosomatic terms to deny access to antimicrobials for systemic infections; and
- force ingestion of psychotropic drugs.

It is the end of financial status determining access to antimicrobial treatment options and persons becoming disabled because they are denied access to generic medicines.

It is the end of sick children under treatment being forcibly removed from their parents and their parents being falsely accused of Munchausen by Proxy.

It is the end of policies and practices that encourage euthanasia and disability over the use of antimicrobials and generic medicines shown to restore the well-being and independence of many thousands.

It is the end of attacks on the human rights defenders of this group. The defenders encompass all medical practitioners and scientific researchers dedicated to ensuring this patient group will enjoy the highest attainable standard of physical and mental health.

It is the end of State actors giving resources to entities and individuals that attack, smear, defame or stigmatize these human rights defenders or the patient group.

It is the end of policies and practices that support of disease-based discrimination and deny human suffering by parsing symptoms, misapplying fraudulent psychosomatic terms to deny medical care and suppressing ethical scientific and medical advances.

It is the end of:
- laws that encourage corruption and drive these abuses;
- government institutions and officials responsible for promoting scientific and medical innovations being patent holders in the same arenas of competition; and
- State actor policies and practices that impoverish patients while enriching private insurers and private medical and scientific investors.

It is also the beginning.

All those concerned with public health, access to health care, scientific advancements that serve the common good, social justice and human dignity need to fully understand this situation.

The human rights abuses experienced by this patient group and their human rights defenders have been institutionalized over the span of four decades and encompass all actors found in modern medical and public health systems.

These abuses are not limited to persons living with Lyme and relapsing fever borreliosis and other coinfections; they encompass more patient groups every day.

These abuses represent trending practices and policies flourishing in systems with weakening accountability and transparency. They are driven by insatiable greed and lack of empathy ... and are boldly corrupting public institutions, elected officials and intergovernmental bodies.

Jenna Luché-Thayer
Founder of the Ad Hoc Committee for Health Equity in ICD11 Borreliosis Codes

Updating ICD11 Borreliosis Diagnostic Codes

Authors are Jenna Luché-Thayer, Holly Ahern, Dominick DellaSala, Sherrill Franklin, Leona Gilbert, Richard Horowitz, Kenneth Liegner, Mualla McManus, Clement Meseko, Judith Miklossy, Natasha Rudenko and Astrid Stuckelberger. Contributing researchers include Joseph Beaton, John Blakely, Phyllis Freeman, Kunal Garg, Huib Kraaijeveld, Vett Lloyd and Leena Meriläinen. Cees Hamelink acted as an Advisor, Jeff Levy provided editorial support and Angelica Johannson provided organizational support. To contact the principal author, email jennaluche@gmail.com

Abstract

This paper analyzes how, on a global scale, existing ICD10 diagnostic codes are preventing proper diagnosis and treatment of borrelioses including Lyme borreliosis and relapsing fever borreliosis. Across the globe, clinicians, scientists, researchers and patients examined and compiled references from peer-reviewed scientific literature to demonstrate the wide-ranging manifestations experienced by patients afflicted with these diseases.

Caused by the bite of ticks, in the United States (US) alone there an estimated 380,000 new annual Lyme borreliosis cases - more cases than breast cancer and more than six times the number of new HIV/AIDS cases.[1] Nevertheless, the few ICD10 diagnostic codes related to the borreliosis illness known Lyme disease cover a fraction of the conditions Lyme disease may cause. On the other hand, several highly unusual and rare conditions currently have their own diagnostic codes including:

W61.62XD	Struck by duck
W55.1	Bitten by a cow
W61.33	Pecked by a chicken
V91.07	Burn due to water skis on fire
V95.40	Unspecified spacecraft accident injuring occupant
R46.1	Bizarre personal appearance

Without accurate and appropriate diagnostic codes, physicians are impeded in their ability to properly care for their patients, leaving those patients invisible and marginalized within the medical system and to those guiding public policy. This results in great personal hardship, pain, disability and expense. This unnecessarily burdens health care systems, governments, families and society as a whole. With accurate diagnostic codes in place, robust data can guide medical and public health research, health policy, track mortality and save health care dollars.

WHO recognizes Lyme disease to be a 'disease of consequence'. WHO has met and consulted with other patient groups, scientists and medical professionals and non-governmental stakeholders from other 'diseases of consequence' during the ICD11 revision process.

We therefore recommend WHO engage with the global borreliosis stakeholder community who recognize the wide-ranging manifestations experienced by borreliosis patients. We also advise WHO use the peer-reviewed scientific literature that recognizes the wide-ranging manifestations experienced by patients as the basis for updating and modernizing the ICD11 diagnostic codes for Lyme borrelioses and relapsing fever borrelioses.

---

[1] Source is the CDC. (2013) International Conference on Lyme Borreliosis and other Tick-borne Diseases. 18 Aug 2013

Edition One: Updating ICD11 Borreliosis Codes

March 29, 2017

Table of Contents

I. Reasons to Update ICD11 Borreliosis Codes — page 1
  I.1. Millions of Persons Made Invisible by ICD10 Borreliosis Codes — page 1
  I.2. ICD10 Borreliosis Codes Generate Flawed Data for Economic
      and Public Health Policy — page 1
      Public Health Policy — page 1
      Sustainable Development Goals — page 2
  I.3. Climate Change is expanding Tick-borne Diseases — page 3
  I.4. ICD10 Borreliosis Codes Undermine WHO's Commitments to Health Equity,
      Human Rights and Gender — page 4
      I.4.1. ICD10 Codes Reinforce Discrimination and Outdated Science
      I.4.2. State-based Human Rights Abuses in Addition to Denial of
      Access to Treatment — page 6
        Sick Children are Taken from Caring Parents — page 6
        Euthanasia is More Reasonable than Generic Antibiotics? — page 7

II. The Understanding of Borreliosis Disease in 2017 — page 8
  II.1. Epidemiology of LB and Relapsing Fever Borreliosis — page 8
  II.2. Phylogeny of LB and Relapsing Fever Borreliosis — page 8
  II.3. LB Pathophysiology, Persistence and Coinfections — page 9
  II.4. Relapsing Fever Borreliosis — page 10
  II.5. Coinfections — page 11

III. Lyme Borreliosis as Obstacle to Healthy Aging — page 11

IV. Reasons for Adapting Borreliosis to be Analogous to Syphilis ICD Codes — page 12
      Existing Diagnostic Codes — page 14

V. Recommendations for ICD Updates for Borreliosis — page 15

VI. Economics, Health and Human Rights — page 17

VII. The ICD11 Beta Platform Exercise — page 20
      Tables of LB Conditions — page 21

VIII. Conclusions — page 53

      Endnotes
      Bibliography
      30 YEARS AND COUNTING

© Copyright 2017. Global Network on Institutional Discrimination
and Ad Hoc Committee for Health Equity in ICD11 Borreliosis Codes
All Rights Reserved

I. Reasons to Update ICD11 Borreliosis Codes

I.1. Millions of Persons Made Invisible by ICD10 Borreliosis Codes

The World Health Organization (WHO) recognizes that vector-borne diseases such as borreliosis are expanding epidemics of global consequence.[1] In the United States (US) alone there an estimated 380,000 new annual Lyme borreliosis cases[2] - more cases than breast cancer and more than six times the number of new HIV/AIDS cases.

In the US, Lyme borreliosis (LB), also referred to as Lyme disease (LD)[3], is the second most common infectious disease tracked by the Centers for Disease Control and Prevention. Rates of the disease are also high in many countries in Europe[4] and China[5] recognizes Lyme borreliosis as the most common tick-borne disease affecting their population.

The existing codes represented in the ICD10 system for LB do not articulate the many common manifestations, stages and complications of LB. ICD10 codes recognize only a limited number of clinical manifestations of disease and are overly focused on the acute form of LB. Furthermore, the ICD10 codes for another spirochete-related disease called "relapsing fever" are not well articulated in the ICD10 system.

Consequently, millions of patients living with complex cases of LB and relapsing fever borreliosis are not represented by the ICD10 codes. Such patients are invisible and are not getting much-needed treatment.

I.2. ICD10 Borreliosis Codes Generate Flawed Data for Economic and Public Health Policy

Public Health Policy

The ICD10 is also a standard statistical instrument. It is used as the basis for comparable statistical data, cause-specific mortality data, morbidity and mortality reporting, general epidemiological purposes, many health management efforts, and the development of sound, rational, cost-effective and humane public health policy. However, because the ICD10 fails to recognize so many clinical manifestations of LB, these statistics are lost.

This has led to (1) public health dollars for Lyme disease being both wasted and insufficiently allocated, resulting on avoidable health care costs and (2) the development of public health policies that appear uncaring and ineffective. Furthermore, the economic impact of these health burdens is unrecognized and uncalculated, in particular in the context of a growing ageing population cumulating overtime an untreated and undiagnosed condition.[6]

> The Centers for Disease Control and Prevention (CDC) estimates US growth of the Lyme disease epidemic to exceed 900 percent.

Nevertheless, the CDC has had no performance metrics to inform policy directed to reduce the human suffering caused by the Lyme disease epidemic.[7]

> For the last four years, the CDC's Lyme disease performance metrics were the establishment of centers that count ticks.

There are no performance metrics related to:
- Reducing the time between infection and diagnosis at all ages
- Improving the treatment options that fail up to 20% percent of diagnosed patients[8]
- Improving screening measures and diagnostic tests that have an approximate accuracy of 50 percent for males and 40 percent accuracy rate for females[9]
- Reducing the growth of the epidemic
- Improving training of health professionals and public health education

Sustainable Development Goals

The United Nations' Sustainable Development Goals (SDG) 2015-2030 include Goal #3 "to ensure healthy lives and promote well-being for all at all ages". The SDG supports the Right to Health;[10] this is a fundamental right enshrined within the international human rights framework reminding us of the imperative of Availability, Accessibility, Acceptability, Quality (AAAQ) of care.[11] The SDG focus on health is as strong as its commitments to economic growth.

There is considerable effort made to collect valid economic data to show gains toward the SDG. For example, "African economies rely heavily on agriculture; for Sub-Saharan Africa, the agriculture sector's share in GDP was 12.7% in 2009, and provided employment to more than 60% of the labor force."[12] Animal husbandry and agriculture are common livelihoods throughout in Africa.

However, economic activities related to animal husbandry and agriculture expose humans to tick-borne pathogens throughout the continent. Among these diseases, tick-borne relapsing fever is caused by several *Borrelia* species. While *B. hermsii*, is the most common cause of relapsing fever in the United States,[13] *B. dutonii* is responsible for the relapsing fever found in central, eastern, and southern Africa.[14] *Borrelia crocidurae* was thought to predominate in West Africa. In fact, two common small mammal reservoirs for *B. crocidurae*, the Guinea multimammate mouse and the African grass rat are commonly found in a wide range of habitats beyond West Africa including Burundi, the Central African Republic, the Democratic Republic of the Congo, Ethiopia, Kenya, Mauritania, the Republic of the Congo, Sudan, and Uganda. The Guinea multimammate mouse's range extends to Cameroon, Morocco and Rwanda and the African grass rat is also found in Eritrea, Malawi, Tanzania, Zambia, Algeria, Egypt, and Yemen.

Furthermore, a 2015 study found 15 tick-borne relapsing borreliosis infected rodent and shrew species common to many areas of Africa.[15] There is obvious risk of exposure to tick-borne relapsing borreliosis through many common agricultural livelihood activities. However, neither the human health or economic impact of relapsing fever borreliosis is routinely or adequately calculated for impact on Sustainable Development Goals in Africa or other areas of the world where relapsing borreliosis and agricultural livelihoods are common.

I.3. Climate Change is expanding Tick-borne Diseases

Tick prevalence, and human tick-borne diseases have significantly increased in the past three decades. Since 2008, climate change and the global response have paved the way for the integration of data on Lyme disease surveillance and vector[16] spread to anticipate human vulnerability to the epidemic.

The consensus of disease ecologists from several countries is that climate change is influencing both abiotic (temperature, humidity levels) and biotic factors (habitat) that contribute to the distribution and reproduction of both hard-body and soft-bodied ticks known to transmit spirochetes to humans. A warming climate and land-use changes are increasing habitat for hosts and creating conditions more favorable for the spread of Lyme borreliosis, particularly in northern latitudes where disease spread and climate change are accelerating.[17]

Climate change is increasing the financial costs and human suffering caused by Lyme borreliosis. The US health care system alone spends an estimated $1.3 billion a year on Lyme borreliosis and these costs will rise as the disease spreads.[18] The impact of the chronic debilitating and disabling form of Lyme borreliosis can destroy human potential, particularly for children, young adults and those vulnerable persons and communities living on the edge of poverty, in poverty, in resource scarce environments and in environments destabilized and degraded by climate change.

I.4. ICD10 Borreliosis Codes Undermine WHO's Commitments to Health Equity, Human Rights and Gender and the fundamental UN Human Right to Health[19]

> "ACCESSIBILITY: Health facilities, goods, and services have to be accessible (physically accessible, affordable, and accessible information) to everyone within the jurisdiction of the State party without discrimination."—WHO principles

When patients with persistent or complicated cases of LB or relapsing fever borreliosis seek medical care, the health service uses a centralized electronic medical information system based upon the ICD10 codes.

However, there are no codes for many forms of borreliosis diseases. Therefore, when a condition found in a certain illness does not match a code, the medical systems that utilize these codes defaults to the 'unspecified illness' category.

If clinical decision support software is utilized, it is based upon the same ICD10 codes, and this software will recommend non-specific 'experimental treatment' for this 'unspecified illness'.

Therefore, treatments for non-acute and many complicated cases of LB and relapsing fever borreliosis are not provided to the patient or limited to those able to afford care that is not covered by insurance and government reimbursements - *this is in opposition to the AAAQ of the Right to Health.*

Those with less disposable income or less power to decide how family resources are allocated, such as women, are particularly vulnerable to lack of access to treatment. Other vulnerable persons challenged by access to treatment include low income and poor women, men and children and the elderly.

> **Obstacles to treatment access can be political.**
>
> In the 1980s, AIDS activists in the US knew many with AIDS were not diagnosed because of the restricted AIDS case definition.
>
> The activists promoted a series of public awareness campaigns including "women don't get AIDS, they just die from it. 65% of HIV positive women get sick and die from chronic infections that don't fit the CDC's definition of AIDS."
>
> Between 1993 and 2016, the AIDS case definition expanded to include more than 60 opportunistic infections.
>
> *Every time the definition expanded, more people gained access to treatment.*

Furthermore, according to a 2008 US government report, Analyses of the Effects of Global Change on Human Health and Welfare and Human Systems,[20] children are considered particularly vulnerable to Lyme disease infection.

I.4.1. ICD10 Codes Reinforce Discrimination and Outdated Science

"The right to health is a fundamental human right that is indispensable for human well-being, for well-functioning societies and economies, and for the ability to exercise all other human rights."[21] WHO 2017

The ICD10 Lyme borreliosis codes are based on outdated science that has been highlighted as a case study in poor practices by the IOM's publication Clinical Practice Guidelines We Can Trust, written in 2011 by the Committee on Standards for Developing Trustworthy Clinical Practice Guidelines.[22]

The case study is found in Chapter 3, page 56, BOX 3-1; it details the lack of transparency regarding the clinical practice guidelines methodologies, particularly with regards to lack of recognition of and treatments for non-acute forms of Lyme disease, e.g. persistent, recurring and complicated forms of the illness.

For most people who have the complicated and persistent forms of LB, the ICD10 Lyme and relapsing fever borreliosis codes result in:

> Today, the situation for millions of Lyme disease patients mirrors the situation endured by HIV/AIDS patients in the 1980s.
>
> Lyme disease patients are told they do not meet the definition of their disease and therefore, they do not deserve treatment.
>
> Unlike AIDS patients, those living with untreated non-acute forms of Lyme disease may linger for decades in severely compromised health and states of disability.
>
> As the immune systems weakens in old age, the illness may emerge and be mistaken as age-related degenerative diseases.
>
> Generic antibiotics can eliminate, reduce or manage many complications of recurring and persistent Lyme disease...
> ... as they do with many recurring and persistent conditions such as acne, rosacea, urinary tract and soft tissue infections.

1. Lack of access and denial of access to treatment options for all stages and complications of relapsing fever and Lyme borreliosis, including persistent LB and other forms of the disease complicated by infection of another tick-borne pathogen and comorbid infections.

2. Denial of the right to informed consent pertaining to full information about the disease and all available treatment.

3. For relapsing fever borreliosis patients, a lack of insurance coverage or government reimbursements for patient-centered treatment options.

4. For LB patients, a lack of insurance coverage or government reimbursements for patient-centered treatment options that meet the Institute of Medicine's (IOM) sanctioned Grading of Recommendations Assessment, Development and Evaluation (GRADE) standards – standards that have been adopted by WHO.[23]

I.4.2. State-based Human Rights Abuses in Addition to Denial of Access to Treatment

Sick Children are Taken from Caring Parents

The ICD codes contribute to other state-based human rights abuses against those living with complicated forms of Lyme borreliosis. In a number of countries, there are many documented cases of government authorities taking children who are sick with Lyme borreliosis away from their parents.

For example, in the Netherlands, an independent organization known as BVIKZ or Interest Group for Intensive Child Care, has undertaken an investigation into false claims of child neglect and abuse by the Dutch Child Protection Services. To date, BVIKZ has compiled and researched 168 individual cases. *Over thirty percent of these cases are about children with Lyme disease.*

Many of these children have the complicated and persistent forms of Lyme borreliosis, or Lyme borreliosis with other coinfections. The degree and duration of the illness often results in children missing school for extended periods of time.

BVIZK compiled a spreadsheet of what is being used as the basis for the allegations. Concerns include many subjective categories such as: 'social isolation', 'cognitive well-being', 'somatic well-being' and 'emotional well-being'. Not going to school for a few weeks is considered as damaging the 'cognitive well-being' of the child and thus framed as 'child abuse'.

According to BVIZK chairman Vera Hooglugt, these situations appear to be subjectively reinterpreted by Dutch Child Protection Services.

> BVIZK chairman Hooglugt observes that "Apparently national Lyme policies dictate that after a few weeks of treatment, the cause of the disease is suddenly a 'mental issue' regardless of the fact that these children are still as ill as before.
>
> Again and again we hear stories of parents who tried everything to get medical help in the Netherlands, but who had to go abroad to find better help." 24
>
> One lawyer has taken up and won three cases on behalf of the parents.
>
> BVIZK chairman Hooglugt thinks that they are only just seeing 'the tip of a much larger iceberg' and wants to encourage other parents to be brave and come with their complaints in case of false allegations.

This short news clip tells part of the story:
https://www.youtube.com/watch?v=RqvXIdO0-Fk

Euthanasia is More Reasonable than Generic Antibiotics?

Teike was a professionally successful, socially well established, and healthy young man until he was bitten by a tick. Teike had a tick bite and the typical rash, Bell's Palsy and other symptoms that indicates an early Lyme borreliosis infection. However, despite sharing this information with medical professionals, he was sent home untested and untreated multiple times from medical centers and emergency rooms after having attacks of severe headaches, light and noise sensitivity, spasms and seizures.

Teike developed serious neurological, arthritic and cardiac symptoms and complications and decided he could wait no longer for diagnosis and treatment. Teike found a medical doctor who is 'BIG-registered' - meaning the doctor meets the criteria to be a registered health professional that is recognized by the Dutch government's Ministry of Health, Welfare and Sport.

This doctor had him tested for tick borne diseases and confirmed he had both Lyme disease and bartonella. Teike responded well to the generic antibiotics commonly used to treat Lyme disease and bartonella, but relapsed after the treatment ended and so he was retreated; he has relapsed again.

In the meanwhile, Teike has found his health insurance company will not cover his treatments with his BIG-registered doctor but will cover a treatment at the Maasstad Hospital. There is an internist and infection specialist at the hospital who offered to treat Teike with 21 days of IV rocephin continued with doxycycline afterwards. However, there is no commitment to treat Teike based upon the severity of his symptoms.

> **The Government's Role in Teike's Case**
>
> The 2002 Dutch Law "Termination of Life on Request and Assisted Suicide Act" states that euthanasia must be undertaken in accordance with criteria of due care. *These criteria note: the patient's suffering - which is supposed to be unbearable and hopeless - and the absence of reasonable alternatives.*
>
> The national government of the Netherlands monitors health access, quality and costs, has responsibility for setting health care priorities, introduces necessary legislative changes related to health care and takes guidance from the National Health Care Institute for defining the statutory benefits package all insurers must provide.
>
> Teike's medical records show his quality of life to be quite bearable when he is treated for his complicated case of Lyme and coinfections. Furthermore, his generic antibiotic treatments follow clinical practices guidelines that meet IOM standards.
>
> Apparently, these IOM sanctioned treatments are not considered to be 'reasonable alternatives' to euthanasia by his insurer Zilveren Kruis (Silver Cross) or the Dutch government.

Teike has expressed that he does not know if he wants to live with this amount of pain and disability. In mid-March 2017, at the age of 29 years old, Teike was told that his insurance company will cover the cost of his euthanasia. [25] See: https://www.youtube.com/watch?v=FoOdSX7wdJ0

II. The Understanding of Borreliosis Disease in 2017

II.1. Epidemiology of LB and Relapsing Fever Borreliosis

Since Lyme arthritis was first noted in the United States in 1977 and the bacterial etiology identified in 1982, the disease has become known as Lyme borreliosis or Lyme disease.[26] The disease was originally labeled "Lyme arthritis" due to the most notable clinical sign among the first cluster of patients studied, swollen knees as a clinical sign of arthritis.[27] In addition to the large joints, and particularly the knee, patients may present with both acute and chronic symptoms affecting the skin, the heart and both the peripheral and central nervous system, vision, digestion, and other systems.

Lyme borreliosis is widely recognized as endemic to the East coast of the United States, Canada, in Europe, Asia, and in China. Relapsing fever borreliosis has a bigger global distribution across Asia, South America, Canada, Australia, Africa, Middle East, Southwestern and Western regions of the USA, and Mexico. Several environmental changes affect the pathogens' prevalence in nature, including climate change and expanding urbanization. These situations are leading to an increasing overlap of human and pathogen reservoirs' habitats.[28]

II.2. Phylogeny of LB and Relapsing Fever Borreliosis

Phylogenetic analysis of the *Borrelia* genus groups the various genospecies into two broad categories: (1) *Borrelia burgdorferi* sensu lato (sl) complex, which accounts for 21 named genospecies, is the most known and studied group; and (2) the relapsing fever group which accounts for nearly 20 genospecies of *Borrelia recurrentis*.[29]

Twenty-one *B. burgdorferi* sl genospecies are recognized and distributed around the world, but new species and variants continue to be recognized. The complex of 21 *Borrelia burgdorferi* genospecies can be divided into two groups based upon the human sensitivity to *B. burgdorferi* sl.[30] They are:

- Ten species with known pathogenicity to humans. This group includes *B. afzelii, B. bavariensis, B. bissettii, B. burgdorferi* sensu stricto, *B. garinii, B. kurtenbachii, B. lusitaniae, B. mayonii, B. spielmanii and B. valaisiana*.

- 11 identified species that have not yet been detected in or isolated from humans. This group includes *B. americana, B. andersonii, B. californiensis, B. carolinensis, B. chilensis, B. finlandensis, B. japonica, B. tanukii, B. turdi, B. sinica, and B. yangtze*.

There is considerable inter- and intra-species diversity among members of these groups, which causes variation in both the clinical presentation of disease and the efficacy of diagnostic tests. The major distinctions between LB and relapsing fever borreliosis are not related to disease manifestations but rather to phylogenetic differences in the *Borrelia* Genus, and the type of vector(s) that are known to transmit the bacteria to humans. Therefore, there is a biological distinction that artificially puts distance between the medical conditions that occur following infection.

Under the existing phylogeny, borreliosis that cause LB are stipulated as being transmitted by "hard-bodied" ticks, only; while those that cause relapsing fever borreliosis are transmitted by either "soft-bodied" ticks or lice. The failure of this classification system is typified by the example of *Borrelia miyamotoi*, a relapsing fever *Borrelia* which is transmitted to humans by the same hard-bodied ticks that transmit *B. burgdorferi* sl to humans.

This is further complicated by the capacity of all kinds of ticks to transmit more than one genospecies of *Borrelia*, and the evolution of new genetic variants of *Borrelia* following infection and dissemination, within a single host.[31]

II.3. LB Pathophysiology, Persistence and Coinfections

Existing scientific evidence indicates that the primary means of transmission of the *B. burgdorferi* sl complex to humans is through a tick bite, the mechanics of which adds a cocktail of immunomodulatory molecules along with the bacteria to prevent inflammation, itching or destruction of the bacteria by the human immune system.

Spirochetes in the *B. burgdorferi* sl complex have developed numerous strategies to further their reproductive agendas, the biomechanics of which are well described in the scientific literature.[32] Survival is achieved by altering the level of gene expression in response to changes in temperature, pH, salts, nutrient content, antibiotic pressure and other host and vector dependent factors.[33]

However, the changes in the genes expression level are not the only route to spirochete survival. Signals that *Borrelia* receives from changing or hostile environments evoke the morphological alterations that keep the pathogen alive and trigger the production of atypical or persistent forms that are refractory to killing by antibiotics.[34]

Starting with exploitation of the immunomodulatory chemicals made by the tick to mask their entry into a new host, the bacteria regulate their gene expression starting early in the infection process[35] and continue through the various stages of dissemination and establishment of permanent colonies called biofilms in various collagen-rich tissues, including the membrane systems of the joints, heart, and nervous system. Once established in biofilms, the infection is tolerant to antibiotic treatment due to protective effects offered by the biofilm. Further antibiotic tolerance is afforded by transformation from metabolic to dormant state, an established bacterial survival mechanism called "persister cells." This is well-established science and has been demonstrated in vitro and in both animal models of Lyme borreliosis and in humans.[36]

It is recognized that the term Lyme borreliosis encompasses a much wider spectrum of diseases for which the etiology had never been established.[37] Lyme borreliosis is a near globally distributed multisystem disorder with a diverse spectrum of clinical manifestations. Many of these clinical manifestations are associated with serious conditions such as multiple sclerosis associated with primary effusion lymphoma,[38] necrotizing granulomatous hepatitis,[39] cutaneous B cell lymphoma[40] and psychiatric disorders[41] or mimic serious conditions such as central nervous system lymphoma.[42]

Disseminated LB can lead to dysregulation across several body systems. As one system becomes dysregulated it may prompt the dysregulation and dysfunction of another system such as endocrine imbalance contributing to immune dysregulation and dysfunction, immune dysregulation and dysfunction contributing to increases in allergies, autoimmune responses and inflammation. Patients with multiple complicating conditions often have associated immune dysfunction.[43] As a result, there is significant variation in disease presentation in those infected with *Borrelia* spp.

II.4. Relapsing Fever Borreliosis

LB has been the primary focus of research on human diseases caused by *Borrelia* genospecies, as illustrated in Table 1. As the returns of the literature search indicates, relapsing fever borreliosis is an under-researched subject in comparison to the existing knowledge base for Lyme borreliosis.

Table 1. Result of PubMed searches pertaining to the terms associated with borreliosis

Search terms used	Number of returned citations
"Borreliosis"	12,311
"Lyme borreliosis"	12,143
"Lyme disease"	11,913
"Relapsing fever"	1881
"Tick-borne relapsing fever"	407
"Louse Borne relapsing fever"	167

Relapsing fever borreliosis generally has an acute onset with non-specific symptoms that can be mistaken for a flu-like viral illness by medical practitioners. Fever can be up to 104 degrees Fahrenheit with associated chills and sweats which can be drenching, which can be confused with other tick-borne infections like babesiosis, Q-fever and brucellosis.

Relapsing fever borreliosis can have associated symptoms of headaches, also seen with infections with *Ehrlichia/Anaplasma* and *C. burnetii*, the myalgias and arthralgias seen with *Ehrlichia*, rickettsial species, and Q fever, as well as the nausea and vomiting that is seen with Rickettsia, *Ehrlichia*, and tick-borne diseases like tularemia in the typhoidal form. Patients may also present with an occasional conjunctivitis and cough.

However, these symptoms are so non-specific that most practitioners would be unable to make the diagnosis unless they have a high level of suspicion and ask about a history of tick-bite.

As in LB, infection with relapsing fever borreliosis has a range of atypical symptoms such as nausea, vomiting, abdominal pain; diarrhea, hepatitis with hepatosplenomegaly and jaundice, which overlap with symptoms associated with Rickettsia.[44]

Relapsing fever borreliosis may also include cardiac manifestations of a myocarditis with arrhythmias, pulmonary symptoms resembling Acute Respiratory Distress Syndrome that is also seen in infection with Babesia species. Other manifestations may include central nervous system manifestations of a facial nerve palsy, hearing loss, iritis, peripheral neuropathy, neuropsychiatric symptoms, stroke with meningoencephalitis and disseminated intravascular coagulation.[45]

II.5. Coinfections

There is a commonly held belief in medicine, called Pasteur's postulate or the Germ Theory, that there is "one cause for one illness" and that bacteria cause acute clinical diseases.

However, exceptions to this simplistic view of the host-pathogen interaction are frequent. Patients with borreliosis are increasingly found to be infected with other microbial pathogens such as *Ehrlichia, Neoehrlichia, Rickettsia, Babesia* and *Theileria* infections which can lead to chronic, rather than acute, illness.[46] Chronic disease symptoms appear more frequently in undiagnosed, untreated, and insufficiently treated patients with borreliosis as well.[47]

Neoehrlichia species is a newly discovered bacterium in ticks and rodents in Europe - Sweden, Switzerland, Germany, and the Czech Republic. It mimics B cell malignancies, and causes non-specific symptoms of fever, muscle and joint pain, vascular and thromboembolic events, including deep vein thrombosis, TIA's, pulmonary embolism, and arterial aneurysms. It can be mistaken for recurrence of hematologic (B cell Lymphomas) or autoimmune diseases and/or unrelated arteriosclerotic vascular events.[48]

III. Lyme Borreliosis as Obstacle to Healthy Aging

Lyme borreliosis also represents a critical obstacle to healthy aging. Due to difficulties in diagnosis and treatment, undiagnosed and untreated tick-borne diseases are often misdiagnosed as chronic inflammatory disorders of aging, that can lead to major age-related degenerative diseases. In certain studies, various spirochetes, absent from healthy brains, are present in 90% of brains of patients with Alzheimer's disease. These spirochetes include Borrelia *burgdorferi*.[49]

Other examples regarding how the disease may be mistaken for age-related illnesses include, but are not limited to cardiac diseases,[50] arthritis,[51] hearing,[52] and vision problems,[53] dementia and Parkinson's disease,[54] strokes,[55] and various psychiatric and gastrointestinal disorders. [56] [57]

Left untreated, Lyme disease can spread and affect almost any part of the body and cause increasing complications with aging. About 60% of untreated patients develop arthritis, which usually affects a knee or other large joint. About 10 - 20% of patients develop neurological or cardiac problems.[59]

It should be noted that some studies indicate that the age of the patients influences the clinical course of borreliosis. Acute and chronic carditis is more common in people aged 16-40 years, whereas neurological disease and arthritis are significantly more common in patients over 40.[60]

In older patients, persistent neurological symptoms including headaches, attention and memory problems, and depression can cumulate over time with polymorbidity and polymedication.

The clinical symptomatology may be mistakenly labelled as "normal pathological ageing" without the consideration of Lyme borreliosis. In such cases, multiple symptoms often mean multiple drugs.

Multiple drugs increase the chances for adverse drug reactions; this possibility for adverse reactions is further increased by the senior ages of the patients.

> **Kris Kristofferson's Lyme disease misdiagnosed as Alzheimer's.[58]**
>
> World famous singer, songwriter and actor Kris Kristofferson's revealed that he was misdiagnosed with Alzheimers. After years of suffering, he tested for positive Lyme disease. His condition improved significantly after just 3 weeks of adequate treatment, making the costly Alzheimers medication and their side effects unnecessary.
>
> According to his wife Lisa "He was taking all these medications for things he doesn't have, and they all have side effects.
>
> "The neurologist suggested anti-seizure medications for passing out, the fibromyalgia doctor was giving him antidepressants for his body pain, his cardiologist gave him a pacemaker for his cardiac arrhythmias, his knees were sore, so he got annual shots from his orthopedist," she said. "It wasn't until I took him to the integrative doctor...that he looked at everything and said, 'This looks like Lyme disease.'
>
> Kristofferson enjoyed many outdoor activities that exposed him to ticks. This risk alone should have prompted an earlier investigation into a possible Lyme disease diagnosis.

IV. Reasons for Adapting Borreliosis to be Analogous to Syphilis ICD Codes

Many of the ICD10 descriptions of syphilis mirror LB complications and these codes can be adapted to represent our understanding of Lyme borreliosis. Many of the ICD10 listings for syphilis have similar counterparts in Lyme borreliosis. Therefore, the ICD10 codes and descriptions for syphilis offer a solid model for the updating of the Lyme borreliosis codes in the ICD11 revision.

Both syphilis and LB have been referred to as the "Great Imitator," because both diseases show great variability in human disease presentations.[61] The similarities between syphilis and Lyme borreliosis have long been recognized among prominent Lyme borreliosis scientists:

> "Although the neurological symptoms and consequences are different, in both diseases (syphilis and Lyme) there are long periods of latent infection in the brain --- followed by a variety of neurological disorders." Dr. Allen C. Steere,
> New York Times, Nov. 22, 1990

> "This disease can involve virtually every organ system of the body. It makes sense to look at this as a whole-body disease, rather than narrowly. In syphilis, which is a similar spirochetes illness in some ways there is also an arthritis. If I concentrated on that aspect of syphilis it would be ludicrous. You wouldn't see the forest for the trees, and I think it's the same thing with this disease." Dr. Raymond Dattwyler
> New York Times, June 12, 1988

> "Lyme disease can produce severe nervous system disorders that look like brain tumors, Alzheimer's disease and multiple sclerosis, sometimes condemning patients to years of needless suffering because of misdiagnosis." Dr. John Halperin
> Chicago Tribune, Sept. 15, 1987

Treponema pallidum, is the spirochetal causative agent of syphilis that has plagued humanity for thousands of years. Both the spirochetal diseases of LB and syphilis can affect multiple organs, demonstrate serovariability over time, and can cause diverse late or chronic manifestations.

Lyme borreliosis, which may be caused by several different genospecies within the *Borrelia* genus, shares many of the same clinical characteristics with syphilis, and the range of human diseases associated with *Borrelia* infections are equally expansive.

However, unlike syphilis, the ICD10 classification system for Lyme borreliosis includes only three codes, for (1) Lyme disease (as defined by the limited case definition for acute Lyme disease); (2) other specified spirochetal infections; and (3) spirochetal infection, unspecified.

The ICD code for relapsing fever, which is dominated by disease states associated with the genospecies *B. duttonii*, does not encompass other relapsing fever borreliosis including that caused by *B. miyomotoi, B. recurrentis, B. hermsii, B. crocidurae*.

For over 25 years, the Lyme borreliosis manifestations that mirror the primary, chronic and late forms of neurosyphilis have been clinically and pathologically confirmed. More than a decade ago, a comprehensive summary of the similar clinical and pathological manifestations found in the different stages of syphilis and Lyme borreliosis was documented in the prestigious Handbook of Clinical Neurology.[62]

Existing Diagnostic Codes

ICD9 and 10 codes for syphilis are extensive and reflect the understanding that syphilis is a complex and potentially devastating disorder with multiple phases, latency, and a wide range of clinical presentations. The same level of awareness and consideration is not afforded to borreliosis, even though both diseases can affect multiple body systems, cause persistent and antibiotic-recalcitrant infections, and lead to chronic diseases that are often medically confused with other disease states.

The ICD9 and 10 codes are inadequate in terms of recognizing the range of *Borrelia* genospecies that cause Lyme disease, the false distinctions between relapsing fever borreliosis and LB based on vector types, and the lack of articulation of LB illness beyond the acute phase.

There are three codes that may cover Lyme borreliosis – A69.2, A69.8 and A69.9. However, any form or manifestation of Lyme borreliosis where the specific *Borrelia* genospecies is not determined, by default reverts to "Lyme disease, unspecified." The other codes are for "other" or "unspecified" disorders, conditions, or spirochetal infections do not include Lyme borreliosis.

There are five subcodes specifically for Lyme disease, that is wrongly described as "an infectious disease caused by a spirochete, *Borrelia burgdorferi*". Furthermore, under code A69.29 the "other conditions associated with Lyme disease" is limited to "Myopericarditis due to Lyme disease". The code A69.20 "Lyme disease unspecified" only describes "Acute Lyme disease and the rash known as Erythema chronica migrans" or bullseye rash.

The codes for Lyme disease's specific conditions are very limited, they are A69.21 "Meningitis due to Lyme disease"; A69.22 "Other neurologic disorders in Lyme disease"; and A69.23 "Arthritis due to Lyme disease". See below.

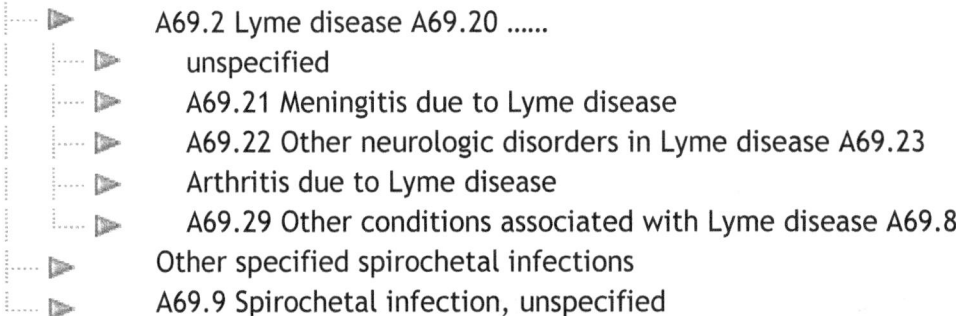

- ▷ A69.2 Lyme disease A69.20 ......
  - ▷ unspecified
  - ▷ A69.21 Meningitis due to Lyme disease
  - ▷ A69.22 Other neurologic disorders in Lyme disease A69.23
  - ▷ Arthritis due to Lyme disease
  - ▷ A69.29 Other conditions associated with Lyme disease A69.8
- ▷ Other specified spirochetal infections
- ▷ A69.9 Spirochetal infection, unspecified

The other codes are for "other" or "unspecified" disorders, conditions, or spirochetal infections. There is no code for latent borreliosis, although latency is well recognized in this disease or the congenital transfer of the disease.[63] There are no codes to specify "Lyme-like" diseases, which are caused *Borrelia* species other than *B. burgdorferi*, such as *B. mayonii*.

Furthermore, the ICD10 only acknowledges the *Borrelia* genospecies of *B. duttonii* that causes relapsing fever. Other *Borrelia* genospecies for relapsing fever require representation such as, *B. crocidurae, B. hispanica, B. duttonii, B. recurrentis* and *B. turicatae*.

V. Recommendations for ICD Updates for Borreliosis

Currently, Lyme borreliosis and relapsing fever borreliosis are interpreted as two unrelated diseases. However, these borrelioses are, in fact, closely related and share similar features. Therefore, given the extensive genetic heterogeneity of the *Borrelia* family, the non-specific and multisystemic nature of symptoms that largely dominate both types of borreliosis, the ICD borreliosis codes should be more integrated and facilitate better characterization of these diseases and their wide range of manifestations.

Poor coding may contribute to misdiagnosis. For example, when the Lyme disease conditions of arthritis and other arthropathies, hearing and vision failure, and neurodegenerative diseases such as dementia and Alzheimer's disease are attributed to aging rather than Lyme disease, the older Lyme disease patient loses the opportunity to reverse and reduce these conditions when treated with antibiotics.

ICD modernization for borreliosis diseases will recognize and integrate advances from scientific research to more accurately reflect the worldwide distribution and range of human illnesses that result from these of diseases. It is recommended that:

1. Revised ICD codes should include a more complete list of the various stages and manifestations of Lyme borreliosis and relapsing fever. For example, ICD codes should reflect that:
   - The immune, endocrine and reticulo-endothelial systems, the skin, the gastrointestinal tract and various organs can all be involved.
   - *Borrelia* infection is found in organic brain syndromes and diverse neurologic manifestations such as seizure disorder, encephalopathy, and a diverse range of neuropsychiatric symptoms.
   - Immunosuppression due to *Borrelial* infection is recognized in the scientific literature, as are *Borrelia*-triggered autoimmune and neuro-autoimmune phenomena.

2. Codes for borreliosis associated with cases of sudden death due to unrecognized Lyme carditis, chronic congestive cardiomyopathies, and chronic and progressive encephalomyelitis including with fatal outcomes, require specific delineation in ICD coding.

3. Model borreliosis codes to reflect the scope and variability of infection, as is done with syphilis coding to include latent, serovariability and seronegative infections. Codes to specify these forms of syphilitic infection exist but are missing for Lyme disease.
   - Just as with syphilis, Lyme borreliosis codes should reflect latency (asymptomatic infection) in early and late stages as well as the serovariability during continuous active infection.

4. Congenital Lyme borreliosis requires clear articulation in the codes.

5. Tick-borne pathogens have been reported in a wide range domestic animals and wildlife reservoirs. There is the need to codify borreliosis - Lyme, Lyme-like and relapsing fever - as zoonoses to guide diagnosis, treatment and prophylaxis, including provisions for recreation and occupational exposures.

6. Many patients with Lyme borreliosis and other tick-borne diseases develop varying degrees of disability, which is sometimes severe. The clinical and laboratory findings that support the recognition of disability from Lyme borreliosis and other tick-borne diseases require attention and articulation in ICD11.

7. Codes should be revised to focus on borreliosis diseases rather than vector sources and revised to accurately reflect multiple vectors of transmission for Pathogens transmitted by body lice or soft-bodied ticks are typically diagnosed as the cause of relapsing fever borreliosis.
   - The ICD10 codes for relapsing fever borreliosis are separate from those that represent Lyme disease. However, these code distinctions are based on the type of louse or tick that transmit the bacteria causing the disease, and not on the clinical presentation of the disease itself which may resemble Lyme disease' or relapsing fever or have symptoms from both.
   - There are relapsing fever borreliosis that include transmission from lice, and hard and soft-bodied ticks.
   - Furthermore, there are indications of hybrid genospecies among the disease causing borreliosis.

8. A single tick bite can result in transmission a multitude of bacterial, viral or protozoal agents. *For this reason, it is vital for the ICD codes to include a code for tick bite, as it does spider bite and insect bite.* In this way, should certain symptoms linked to tickborne illnesses manifest, medical records will link back to the tick bite incident and assist with arriving at the proper diagnosis.

9. A number of un-coded conditions that may be caused by borreliosis should be properly noted under those conditions; as is found under the ICD10 code G01 "Meningitis in bacterial diseases classified elsewhere".

10. There are other tick-borne diseases, while not addressed within the scope of this paper, that deserve more articulation of their manifestations and be updated in the ICD11 by WHO.

ICD10

G01 Meningitis in bacterial diseases classified elsewhere

- meningitis (in):
- gonococcal (A54.81)
- leptospirosis (A27.81)
- listeriosis (A32.11)
- Lyme disease (A69.21)
- meningococcal (A39.0)
- neurosyphilis (A52.13)
- tuberculosis (A17.0)

The following recommendations are related to the broader mandates of WHO

11. The lack of support for borreliosis research in sub Saharan Africa is reflected in under-reporting and skewed global prevalence rates. There should be effort made to improve surveillance and study of these diseases in this region.

12. There should be a concerted effort to make provisions for inclusion of Borrelia in differential diagnoses for malaria, dengue, lassa and other fevers of unknown etiology in sub Saharan Africa. This would ensure patients with clinical borreliosis are not excluded from treatment due to missed diagnoses.

13. Governmental travel guidance should integrate accurate health warnings for travelers in the countries and regions under the wide global range of borreliosis.

14. Questions on travel history should be integrated into the medical and clinical reviews of patients.

15. Studies beyond the acute presentation of borreliosis are required to investigate the biological basis for the clinical disease variability observed in humans. For example, there is significant variation in disease presentation, which is likely due to a combination of various factors influencing pathogen-host interactions, including the virulence of the infecting *Borrelia* genospecies, the age, the genetic predisposition, and the immune status of the host.

16. There is the ongoing need to find promising treatments from antibiotic combinations and non-antibiotic treatments and to increase understanding regarding the transmission of borreliosis infection by other biting insects, blood transfusions, organ transplants and possible sexual transmission.

VI. Economics, Health and Human Rights

WHO's Constitution defines health as 'a state of complete physical, mental and social well-being and not merely the absence of disease or infirmity.' Therefore, any remaining reasons to continue with these inadequate LB codes wither before the human rights' protections they violate.[64]

WHO acts in compliance with the Committee on Economic, Social and Cultural Rights and Social Council (ECOSOC) and the International Covenant on Economic, Social and Cultural Rights (ICESCR) – Article 12. Excerpts from ICESCR's Health and Human Rights follow. The Covenant recognizes the right of everyone to achieve the highest attainable standard of physical and mental health. Steps to be taken to achieve the full realization of this right shall include those necessary for:
- the prevention, treatment and control of epidemic, endemic, occupational and other diseases
- the creation of conditions which would assure to all medical service and medical attention in the event of sickness.

Access to medicines is an integral part of the right to health and covered by the core obligations of the rights to health. A table detailing the 'Impact of Current ICD LB Codes on Health and Human Rights' now follows.

Impact of Current ICD LB Codes on Health and Human Rights	
Health and Human Rights	Impact of ICD LB Codes on all persons who develop non-acute forms of LB by living and travelling in member states where the codes have been adopted
Availability: Functioning public health and healthcare facilities, goods, services and programs must be available in sufficient quantity	Current ICD LB codes limit availability of IOM sanctioned treatment protocols to those persons able to pay for their medication independently of government and/or insurance coverage
Accessibility: Health facilities, goods and services must be accessible to everyone without discrimination	LB patients with non-acute forms of the disease are discriminated against, those persons unable to pay for their medication independently of government and/or insurance coverage are greatly disadvantaged.
Information accessibility: The right to seek, receive and impart information and ideas concerning health issues.	LB patients with the non-acute LB are routinely denied information regarding treatment options found in IOM sanctioned clinical guidelines, their forms of LB are largely ignored by WHO and many governmental institutions. The LB stakeholder group is routinely denied engagement opportunities - *readily provided to other stakeholder groups* - to impart information and ideas concerning LB health issues.
Acceptability means all health facilities, goods and services are respectful of medical ethics.	The evidence of code-based discrimination makes for the appearance of limited application of medical ethics.
All services are scientifically and medically appropriate and of good quality	'Quality' is limited to the acute form of the disease as the current codes ignore much relevant science and medical knowledge.
The right to health imposes the obligations to respect, protect and fulfil.	
Refrain from interfering directly or indirectly with the enjoyment of the right to health	Current codes interfere directly and indirectly with this right by reducing access to treatments and treatment options across all member states that have adopted the codes
Prevent third parties from interfering these guarantees of health rights	There have been indications of interference by third parties, but more information is required to determine this matter

The logic, objectives and benefits of changing these borreliosis codes must be obvious to many public health professionals, most economists, medical practitioners and social scientists. In addition to sound scientific and medical reasons, there are economic and humanitarian reasons for updating the codes. The table below provides a summary of such reasons.

Inadequate versus Updated Lyme Borreliosis Codes	
The information provided in this table conforms to WHO's commitment to the Rational Use of Medicines [65] wherein WHO advocates 12 key interventions to promote more rational use including *"the use of clinical guidelines, the use of independent information on medicines and the avoidance of perverse financial incentives".*	
OUTCOMES **Current LB ICD Codes**	**OUTCOMES** **With Updated LB ICD Codes**
In the US for-profit medical system, an undiagnosed, or diagnosed and under-treated, Lyme disease patient can easily generate hundreds of thousands of dollars in profits for pharmaceutical, research and medical interests peddling expensive patented drugs designed to provide some relief and a dependence of life long maintenance, and medical devices that replace knees and hips ravaged by chronic infection. Many of these persons become unemployable. Those who become unemployed, or survive beyond their insurance benefits, will then drain tax dollars set aside for the medical care of the poor and elderly.	IOM sanctioned clinical guidelines and treatment protocols using inexpensive generic drugs may eliminate, reduce or manage LB in its acute, disseminated, complicated and chronic forms. Such drugs and protocols are routinely and safely used for a wide a variety of diseases by many patient groups throughout the world. Many LB patients under patient-centered protocols are able to continue in school and work, provide and care for their families, and contribute resources and time to their communities.
Inadequate LB ICD codes defeat public health policy objectives and threaten reserves set aside for the poor and elderly.	Updated LB ICD codes support improved well-being, functional independence, productivity and financial health.

VII. The ICD11 Beta Platform Exercise

In response to the February 27, 2017 request by Dr. Ian Smith, Executive Director for the Office of the Director-General of WHO, the Ad Hoc Committee for Health Equity in ICD11 Borreliosis Codes 'further refined the recommendations' submitted in their February 2017 draft <u>Updating the ICD11 Borreliosis Codes</u> report. As requested by Dr. Smith, The Ad Hoc Committee also, 'provided greater specificity with regards to the proposed codes relating to Borreliosis infection and submitted them into the ICD11 Beta Platform. This specificity can be verified by comparing the earlier recommendations (see pages 15 -17) to the ensuing tables.

It must be noted that many persons in the global borreliosis community vounteered to submit the Ad Hoc committee's updated proposals for the borreliosis codes onto the ICD11 Beta Platform. Most of these persons were Lyme patients, caretakers and advocates and many have university degrees and professional standing. However, many were unable to navigate the ICD11 Beta Platform. They then co-authored a letter to document their experience and submitted the letters independently to WHO from their countries. Excerpts from this letter follow:

> "In the video...Dr. Kieny invited all stakeholders to participate in the ICD11 Beta Platform. Therefore, I registered on the ICD11 Beta Platform to submit proposals for Lyme borreliosis. I wanted to add Lyme borreliosis conditions and complications that are not found in the ICD10 codes...However, I was not able to use your ICD11 Beta Platform; it is too complicated. I am not a clinician or expert in information technology...
>
> I understand that ... at the Tokyo ICD-11 revision conference, Dr. Margaret Chan, Director-General of WHO said, "This has been the most challenging, complex, and far-reaching ICD revision in the 100-year history of this standard statistical instrument." She also said, "thousands of clinicians and experts in information technology have contributed to this comprehensive revision."
>
> I also understand that WHO has spent money training persons on how to use small portions of the ICD codes and the related information systems; I wish you had trained me to use this system. I wish I - or anyone I know who lives with complicated and persistent Lyme borreliosis - had been invited to your many ICD11 revision stakeholder events. I want to be a stakeholder in the ICD11 revision process; but I have been excluded by your lack of invitation to any of the ICD11 revision stakeholder events and a Beta Platform that was not designed for use by the average stakeholder.
>
> I do not understand why you would allow for codes that only recognize a fraction of the Lyme borreliosis complications and result in denial of treatment. Your codes are taking away the future of children who are sick with this disease. This makes no sense when generic drugs can be used to eliminate, reduce and manage symptoms and persistent infection. This is very cruel and feels like discrimination."

Tables of LB Conditions

The Ad Hoc Committee submitted each manifestation noted the following tables. We anticipate there will be need for clarification and revisions and we understand there are extensive opportunities for post-coordination in ICD-11.

Some definitions of Terminology

- ✓ The secondary stage results from the dissemination of Borrelia during the early latent stage.
- ✓ The late stage is considered chronic if the duration is more than six months.
- ✓ ** (double red asterisks) indicates possibility of fatality from the condition

TABLE 1 Congenital Lyme

Congenital Lyme disease	References
Borrelia burgdorferi can potentially infect the fetus and cause adverse fetal outcomes **	Bale JF, Murph JR. Congenital infections and the nervous system. *Pediatric Clinics of North America*. 1992;39(4):669-690. doi:10.1016/s0031-3955(16)38370-5. [PubMed] Brzostek T. [Human granulocytic ehrlichiosis co-incident with Lyme borreliosis in pregnant woman--a case study] [in Polish] *Przegl Epidemiol*. 2004;58(2):289-94. [PubMed] Gardner T. Lyme disease. In: Remington JS, Klein JO, eds. *Infectious Diseases of the Fetus and Newborn*. 5th ed. Philadelphia: Saunders; 1995:447-528chap 11. Gardner T. Lyme disease. In: Remington JS, Klein JO. *Infectious diseases of the fetus and newborn infant*. 4th ed. Philadelphia: W B Saunders Co; December 13, 1994. Goldenberg RL, Thompson C. The infectious origins of stillbirth. *American Journal of Obstetrics and Gynecology*. 2003;189(3):861-873. doi:10.1067/s0002-9378(03)00470-8. [PubMed] Gustafson JM, Burgess EC, Wachal MD, Steinberg H. Intrauterine transmission of Borrelia burgdorferi in dogs. *American Journal of Veterinary Research*. 1993;54(6):882-890. [PubMed]

Congenital Lyme disease	References
	MacDonald AB, Benach JL, Burgdorfer W. Stillbirth following maternal Lyme disease. *N Y State J Med*. 1987;11:615-616. [PubMed]

MacDonald AB. Gestational Lyme borreliosis. Implications for the fetus. *Rheum Dis Clin North Am*. 1989;15(4):657-677. [PubMed]

Macdonald AB. Human fetal borreliosis, toxemia of pregnancy, and fetal death. *Zentralblatt für Bakteriologie, Mikrobiologie und Hygiene. Series A: Medical Microbiology, Infectious Diseases, Virology, Parasitology*. 1986;263(1-2):189-200. doi:10.1016/s0176-6724(86)80122-5. [PubMed]

Maraspin V, Cimperman J, Lotric-Furlan S, Pleterski-Rigler D, Strle F. Erythema migrans in pregnancy. *Wiener klinische Wochenschrift*. 2000;111:933-40. [PubMed]

Markowitz LE, Steere AC, Benach JL, Slade JD, Broome CV. Lyme disease during pregnancy. *JAMA: The Journal of the American Medical Association*. 1986;255(24):3394. doi:10.1001/jama.1986.03370240064038. PubMed

Schlesinger PA, Duray PH, Burke BA, Steere AC, Stillman MT. Maternal-fetal transmission of the Lyme disease Spirochete, Borrelia burgdorferi. *Annals of Internal Medicine*. 1985;103(1):67. doi:10.7326/0003-4819-103-1-67. [PubMed]

Silver RM, Yang L, Daynes RA, Branch WD, Salafia CM, Weis JJ. Fetal outcome in Murine Lyme disease. *Infection and Immunity*. 1995;63(1):66-72. [PubMed]

Strobino BA, Williams CL, Abid S, Ghalson R, Spierling P. Lyme disease and pregnancy outcome: A prospective s of two thousand prenatal patients. *American Journal of Obstetrics and Gynecology*. 1993;169(2):367-374. doi:10.1016/0002-9378(93)90088-z. [PubMed]

Weber K, Bratzke H-J, Neubert U, Wilske B, Duray PH. Borrelia burgdorferi in a newborn despite oral penicillin for Lyme borreliosis during pregnancy. *The Pediatric Infectious Disease Journal*. 1988;7(4):286-288. doi:10.1097/00006454-198804000-00010. [PubMed] |

TABLE 2 Primary Infection & Erythema migrans

	References
Primary infection - Erythema migrans	Christova I, Komitova R. Clinical and epidemiological features of Lyme borreliosis in Bulgaria. Wien Klin Wochenschr. 2004;116(1-2):42-6. [PubMed] Hercogová J, Tománková M, Barták P. Contributions to the treatment of dermatologic manifestations of Lyme borreliosis. Cutis. 1992 Jun;49(6):409-11. [PubMed] Lipsker D, Hansmann Y, Limbach F, Clerc C, Tranchant C, Grunenberger F, Caro-Sampara F, Attali P, Frey M, Kubina M, Piémont Y, Sibilia J, Jaulhac B; GEBLY Study Group. Study Group for Lyme Borreliosis. Disease expression of Lyme borreliosis in northeastern France. Eur J Clin Microbiol Infect Dis. 2001;20(4):225-30. [PubMed] Melski JW, Reed KD, Mitchell PD, Barth GD. Primary and secondary erythema migrans in central Wisconsin. Arch Dermatol. 1993;129(6):709-16. [PubMed] Schmid GP. Epidemiology and clinical similarities of human spirochetal diseases. Rev Infect Dis. 1989;11Suppl 6:S1460-9. Review type. [PubMed]
Primary Infection, seronegative Early Lyme disease 'seronegative' is not a 'separate condition' - it is an aspect of the disease recognizing patients may test negative when infected.	Coyle PK, Deng Z, Schutzer SE, Belman AL, Benach J, Krupp LB, Luft B. Detection of Borrelia burgdorferi antigens in cerebrospinal fluid. Neurology 1993;43:1093-1097. [PubMed] Coyle PK, Schutzer SE, Deng Z, et al. Detection of Borrelia burgdorferi-specific antigen in antibody-negative cerebrospinal fluid in neurologic Lyme disease. Neurology. 1995;45(11):2010-2015. [PubMed] Dattwyler RJ, Volkman DJ, Luft BJ, Halperin JJ, Thomas J, Golightly MG. Seronegative Lyme Disease. Dissociation of T- and B-Lymphocyte Responses to Borrelia burgdorferi. N Engl J Med 1988;319:1441-6. [PubMed] Holak H1, Holak N, Huzarska M, Holak S. Tick inoculation in an eyelid region: report on five cases with one complication of the orbital myositis associated with Lyme borreliosis. Klin Oczna. 2006;108(4-6):220-4. [PubMed] Karma A, Seppälä I, Mikkilä H, Kaakkola S, Viljanen M, Tarkkanen A. Diagnosis and clinical characteristics of ocular Lyme borreliosis. Am J Ophthalmol. 1995;119(2):127-35. [PubMed] Lawrence C, Lipton RB, Lowy FD, Coyle PK. Seronegative Chronic Relapsing Neuroborreliosis. Eur Neurol 1995;35:113-117. [PubMed]

TABLE 3 Persistent Infection in Secondary & Late Stages

Persistent infection	References
	Feng J., Wang T., Shi W., Zhang S., Sullivan D., Auwaerter P.G., Zhang Y. Identification of novel activity against Borrelia burgdorferi persisters using an FDA approved drug library. Emerg. Microbes Infect. 2014;3:e49. doi: 10.1038/emi.2014.53. [PMC free article] [PubMed] [Cross Ref] Oksi J., Marjamaki M., Nikoskelainen J., Viljanen M.K. *Borrelia burgdorferi* detected by culture and PCR in clinical relapse of disseminated Lyme borreliosis. Ann. Med. 1999;31:225-232. doi: 10.3109/07853899909115982. [PubMed] [Cross Ref] Preac-Mursic V, Pfister HW, Spiegel H, Burk R, Wilske B, Reinhardt S, Bohmer R. First Isolation of Borrelia burgdorferi from an Iris Biopsy. J Clin Neuro-ophthalmol 1993;13:155-161. [PubMed] Preac-Mursic V, Weber K, Pfister HW, Wilske B, Gross B, Baumann A, Prokop J. Survival of Borrelia burgdorferi in Antibiotically Treated Patients with Lyme borreliosis. Infection 1989;17:355-359. [PubMed] Schmidli J., Hunziker T., Moesli P., Schaad U.B. Cultivation of *Borrelia burgdorferi* from joint fluid three months after treatment of facial palsy due to Lyme borreliosis. J. Infect. Dis. 1988;158:905-906. doi: 10.1093/infdis/158.4.905. [PubMed] [Cross Ref]

TABLE 4 Secondary and Late infection - Cutaneous

Borrelial lymphocytoma (BL)	References
	Arnež M, Ružić-Sabljić E. Borrelial Lymphocytoma in Children. Pediatr Infect Dis J. 2015;34(12):1319-22. [PubMed] Colli C, Leinweber B, Müllegger R, Chott A, Kerl H, Cerroni L. Borrelia burgdorferi-associated lymphocytoma cutis: clinicopathologic, immunophenotypic, and molecular study of 106 cases. J Cutan Pathol. 2004;31(3):232-40. [PubMed] Glatz M, Resinger A, Semmelweis K, Ambros-Rudolph CM, Müllegger RR. Clinical spectrum of skin manifestations of Lyme borreliosis in 204 children in Austria. Acta Derm Venereol. 2015;95(5):565-71. [PubMed] Gordillo-Pérez G, Torres J, Solórzano-Santos F, de Martino S, Lipsker D, Velázquez E, Ramon G, Onofre M, Jaulhac B. Borrelia burgdorferi infection and cutaneous Lyme disease, Mexico. Emerg Infect Dis. 2007;13(10):1556-8. [PubMed] Krbkova L, Stanek G. Therapy of Lyme borreliosis in children. Infection. 1996;24(2):170-3. [PubMed] Lenormand C, Jaulhac B, De Martino S, Barthel C, Lipsker D. Species of Borrelia burgdorferi complex that cause borrelial lymphocytoma in France. Br J Dermatol. 2009;161(1):174-6. [PubMed] Maraspin V, Cimperman J, Lotric-Furlan S, Ružić-Sabljić E, Jurca T, Picken RN, Strle F. Solitary borrelial lymphocytoma in adult patients. Wien Klin Wochenschr. 2002;114(13-14):515-23. [PubMed] Maraspin V, Nahtigal Klevišar M, Ružić-Sabljić E, Lusa L, Strle F. Borrelial Lymphocytoma in Adult Patients. Clin Infect Dis. 2016;63(7):914-21. [PubMed] Müllegger RR, Means TK, Shin JJ, Lee M, Jones KL, Glickstein LJ, Luster AD, Steere AC. Chemokine signatures in the skin disorders of Lyme borreliosis in Europe: predominance of CXCL9 and CXCL10 in erythema migrans and acrodermatitis and CXCL13 in lymphocytoma. Infect Immun. 2007;75(9):4621-8. [PubMed] Strle F, Maraspin V, Pleterski-Rigler D, Lotric-Furlan S, Ružić-Sabljić E, Jurca T, Cimperman J. Treatment of borrelial lymphocytoma. Infection. 1996;24(1):80-4. [PubMed]

Acrodermatitis atrophicans	**References** Aberer E, Klade H. Cutaneous manifestations of Lyme borreliosis. Infection. 1991 Jul-Aug;19(4):284-6. [PubMed] Busch U, Hizo-Teufel C, Böhmer R, Fingerle V, Rössler D, Wilske B, Preac-Mursic V. Borrelia burgdorferi sensu lato strains isolated from cutaneous Lyme borreliosis biopsies differentiated by pulsed-field gel electrophoresis. Scand J Infect Dis. 1996;28(6):583-9. [PubMed] Schempp C, Bocklage H, Lange R, Kölmel HW, Orfanos CE, Gollnick H. Further evidence for Borrelia burgdorferi infection in morphea and lichen sclerosus et atrophicus confirmed by DNA amplification. J Invest Dermatol. 1993;100(5):717-20. [PubMed] Wienecke R1, Zöchling N, Neubert U, Schlüpen EM, Meurer M, Volkenandt M. Molecular subtyping of Borrelia burgdorferi in erythema migrans and acrodermatitis chronica atrophicans. J Invest Dermatol. 1994;103(1):19-22. [PubMed]
Granuloma annulare, morphea, localized scleroderma, lichen sclerosus & atrophicus	Aberer E, Schmidt BL, Breier F, Kinaciyan T, Luger A. Amplification of DNA of Borrelia burgdorferi in urine samples of patients with granuloma annulare and lichen sclerosus et atrophicus. 1999;135(2):210-2. [PubMed] Asbrink E, Brehmer-Andersson E, Hovmark A. Acrodermatitis chronica atrophicans--a spirochetosis. Clinical and histopathological picture based on 32 patients; course and relationship to erythema chronicum migrans Afzelius. Am J Dermatopathol. 1986;8(3):209-19. [PubMed] Buechner SA, Winkelmann RK, Lautenschlager S, Gilli L, Rufli T. Localized scleroderma associated with Borrelia burgdorferi infection. Clinical, histologic, and immunohistochemical observations. J Am Acad Dermatol. 1993;29(2 Pt 1):190-6. [PubMed] Eisendle K, Grabner T, Zelger B. Morphoea: a manifestation of infection with Borrelia species? Br J Dermatol. 2007;157(6):1189-98. [PubMed] Kaya G, Berset M, Prins C, Chavaz P, Saurat JH. Chronic borreliosis presenting with morphea- and lichen sclerosus et atrophicus-like cutaneous lesions. a case report. Dermatology. 2001;202(4):373-5. [PubMed] Malane MS, Grant-Kels JM, Feder HM Jr, Luger SW. Diagnosis of Lyme disease based on dermatologic manifestations. Ann Intern Med. 1991;114(6):490-8. [PubMed]

Granuloma annulare, morphea, localized scleroderma, lichen sclerosus & atrophicus	References Menni S, Pistritto G, Gelmetti C, Stanta G, Trevisan G. Eruzione a tipo pitiriasi lichenoide con perifolliculiti in corso di borreliosi di Lyme. Eur J Pediat Dermatol. 1994;4:77-80. Ozkan S, Atabey N, Fetil E, Erkizan V, Günes AT. Evidence for Borrelia burgdorferi in morphea and lichen sclerosus. Int J Dermatol. 2000;39(4):278-83. [PubMed] Schempp C, Bocklage H, Lange R, Kölmel HW, Orfanos CE, Gollnick H. Further evidence for Borrelia burgdorferi infection in morphea and lichen sclerosus et atrophicus confirmed by DNA amplification. J Invest Dermatol. 1993;100(5):717-20. [PubMed] Trevisan G, Rees DH, Stinco G. Morphea Borrelia burgdorferi and localized scleroderma. Clin Dermatol. 1994;12(3):475-9. [ScienceDirect] Vasudevan B, Chatterjee M. Lyme Borreliosis and Skin. Indian J Dermatol. 2013;58(3): 167-174. doi: 10.4103/0019-5154.110822 [PubMed] Vasudevan B, Sagar A, Bahal A, Mohanty AP. Extragenital lichen sclerosus with aetiological link to Borrelia. MJAFI. 2011;67:370-3. [PubMed] Zinchuk AN, Kalyuzhna LD, Pasichna IA. Is Localized Scleroderma Caused by Borrelia burgdorferi? Vector Borne Zoonotic Dis. 2016;16(9):577-80. [PubMed]
Other cutaneous manifestations	Abele DC, Anders KH, Chandler FW. Benign lymphocytic infiltration (Jessner-Kanof): another manifestation of borreliosis? *J Am Acad Dermatol.* 1989;21(4 Pt 1):795-7. [PubMed] Baldari U, Cattonar P, Nobile C, Celli B, Righini MG, Trevisan G. Infantile acrodermatitis of Gianotti-Crosti and Lyme borreliosis. *Acta Derm Venereol.* 1996;76(3):242-3. [PubMed] Hashimoto Y, Takahashi H, Matsuo S, Hirai K, Takemori N, Nakao M, Miyamoto K, Iizuka H. Polymerase chain reaction of Borrelia burgdorferi flagellin gene in Shulman syndrome. *Dermatology.* 1996;192(2):136-9. [PubMed] Lesire V, Machet L, Toledano C, de Muret A, Maillard H, Lorette G, Vaillant L. Atypical erythema multiforme occurring at the early phase of Lyme disease? *Acta Derm Venereol.* 2000;80(3):222. [PubMed] Olson JC, Esterly NB. Urticarial vasculitis and Lyme disease. *J Am Acad Dermatol.* 1990;22(6 Pt 1):1114-6. [PubMed]

Lyme disease of skin and mucous membranes	**References** Asbrink E, Hovmark A. Lyme borreliosis: aspects of tick-borne Borrelia burgdorferi infection from a dermatologic viewpoint. *Semin Dermatol.* 1990;9(4):277-91. [PubMed] Middelveen MJ, Bandoski C, Burke J, Sapi E, Filush KR, Wang Y, Franco A, Mayne P, Stricker RB. Exploring the association between Morgellons disease and Lyme disease: identification of Borrelia burgdorferi in Morgellons disease patients. BMC Dermatol. 2015 Feb 12;15:1. [PubMed] Vasudevan B, Chatterjee M. Lyme Borreliosis and Skin. *Indian J Dermatol.* 2013; 58(3):167-174. [PubMed]
Lyme alopecia	Cimperman J, Maraspin V, Lotric-Furlan S, Ruzić-Sabljić E, Avsic-Zupanc T, Strle F. Diffuse reversible alopecia in patients with Lyme meningitis and tick-borne encephalitis. *Wiener klinische Wochenschrift.* 2000;111:976-7. [PubMed] Gubertini N, Bonin S, Trevisan G. Lichen sclerosus et atrophicans, scleroderma en coup de sabre and Lyme borreliosis. *Dermatol Reports.* 2011;28;3(2):e27. doi: 10.4081/dr.2011.e27. [PubMed] Hercogová J, Brzonova I. Lyme disease in central Europe. *Curr Opin Infect Dis.* 2001;14(2):133-7. [PubMed] Schwarzenbach R, Djawari D. [Pseudopelade Brocq--possible sequela of stage III borrelia infection?] [in German]. *Der Hautarzt; Zeitschrift fur Dermatologie, Venerologie, und verwandte Gebiete.* 1999;49(11):835-7. [PubMed]
Other lesions in Lyme disease	Bauer J1, Leitz G, Palmedo G, Hügel H. Anetoderma: another facet of Lyme disease? *J Am Acad Dermatol.* 2003;48(5 Suppl):S86-8. [PubMed] Glatz M, Resinger A, Semmelweis K, Ambros-Rudolph CM, Müllegger RR. Clinical spectrum of skin manifestations of Lyme borreliosis in 204 children in Austria. *Acta Derm Venereol.* 2015;95(5):565-71. [PubMed] Melski JW, Reed KD, Mitchell PD, Barth GD. Primary and secondary erythema migrans in central Wisconsin. *Arch Dermatol.* 1993;129(6):709-16. [PubMed]

TABLE 5 Secondary and late Lyme meningitis, oculopathy, iridocyclitis, iritis, uveitis

Lyme meningitis **	References
	Bingham PM, Galetta SL, Athreya B, Sladky J. Neurologic manifestations in children with Lyme disease. Pediatrics. 1995;96:1053-1056. [PubMed]
	Ginsberg L, Kidd D. Chronic and recurrent meningitis. Pract Neurol. 2008 Dec;8(6):348-61. Review doi: 10.1136/jnnp.2008.157396. [PubMed]
	Pachner AR. Early disseminated Lyme disease: Lyme meningitis. Am J Med. 1995 Apr 24;98(4A):30S-37S; discussion 37S-43S. [PubMed]
	Steere AC, Bartenhagen NH, Craft JE, Hutchinson GJ, Newman JH, Pachner AR, Rahn DW, Sigal LH, Taylor E, Malawista SE. Clinical manifestations of Lyme disease. *Zentralbl Bakteriol Mikrobiol Hyg A*. 1986;263(1-2):201-5.[PubMed]
Lyme oculopathy	Karma A, Seppälä I, Mikkilä H, Kaakkola S, Viljanen M, Tarkkanen A. Diagnosis and clinical characteristics of ocular Lyme borreliosis. *Am J Ophthalmol*. 1995;119(2):127-35. doi:10.1016/s0002-9394(14)73864-4. [PubMed]
	Mikkilä HO, Seppala IJ, Viljanen MK, Peltomaa MP, Karma A. The expanding clinical spectrum of ocular lyme borreliosis. *Ophthalmology* 2000;107:581-587. [PubMed]
	Raja H, Starr MR, Bakri SJ. Ocular manifestations of tick-borne diseases. *Surv Ophthalmol*. 2016;61(6):726-744. Review. doi: 10.1016/j.survophthal.2016.03.011. [PubMed]
	Sathiamoorthi S, Smith WM. The eye and tick-borne disease in the United States. *Curr Opin Ophthalmol*. 2016;27(6):530-537. Review. DOI: 10.1097/ICU.0000000000000308 [PubMed]
Lyme iridocyclitis, iritis	Boutros A, Rahn E, Nauheim R. Iritis and papillitis as a primary presentation of Lyme disease. *Ann Ophthalmol*. 1990;22(1):24-5. [PubMed]
	Golubić D, Vinković T, Turk D, Hranilović J, Slugan I. [Ocular manifestations of Lyme borreliosis in northwest Croatia]. Lijec Vjesn. 2004;126(5-6):124-8. [Article in Croatian] [PubMed]
	Winward KE, Smith JL, Culbertson WW, Paris-Hamelin A. Ocular Lyme borreliosis. *Am J Ophthalmol*. 1989;15;108(6):651-7. [PubMed]

Lyme uveitis	**References** Isogai E, Isogai H, Kotake S, Yoshikawa K, Ichiishi A, Kosaka S, Sato N, Hayashi S, Oguma K, Ohno S. Detection of antibodies against Borrelia burgdorferi in patients with uveitis. *Am J Ophthalmol*. 1991;15;112(1):23-30. [PubMed] Marguet C, Rouillier-Saas M, Mallet E, Meunier M, Jeannot E, Boulloche J, Forget C. [Lyme disease in Upper Normandy: report of a hospital survey]. *Arch Pediatr*. 2000;7 Suppl 3:517s-522s. French. [PubMed] Veyssier P. [Clinical manifestations of Lyme disease]. Rev Prat. 1989; 18;39(15):1294-9. French [PubMed]

TABLE 6 Secondary & Late Lyme nephritis, hepatitis, lymphadenopathy, myositis & other

Lyme nephritis **	References
	Kelly B, Finnegan P, Cormican M, Callaghan J. Lyme disease and glomerulonephritis. *Ir Med J*. 2017;92(5):372. [PubMed] Kirmizis D, Chatzidimitriou D. Comment on 'Membranous glomerulonephritis secondary to Borrelia burgdorferi infection presenting as nephrotic syndrome'. *Nephrology Dialysis Transplantation*. 2010;25(5):1723-1727. doi:10.1093/ndt/gfq028. [PubMed] Kirmizis D, Chatzidimitriou D. Renal Manifestations of Lyme Disease: Interplay between Infection and Immunostimulation. In: Holmgren A, Borg G, ed. *Handbook Of Disease Outbreaks: Prevention, Detection And Control*. 1st ed. New York: Nova Science Publishers Inc; 2010. [https://www.novapublishers.com/catalog/product_info.php?products_id=11009] Kirmizis D, Efstratiadis G, Economidou D, Diza-Mataftsi E, Leontsini M, Memmos D. MPGN secondary to lyme disease. *American Journal of Kidney Diseases*. 2004;43(3):544-551. doi:10.1053/j.ajkd.2003.11.014. [PubMed] Kwiatkowska E, Gołembiewska E, Ciechanowski K, Kędzierska K. Minimal-Change Disease Secondary toBorrelia burgdorferiInfection. *Case Reports in Nephrology*. 2012;2012:1-3. doi:10.1155/2012/294532. [PubMed] Mc Causland F, Niedermaier S, Bijol V, Rennke H, Choi M, Forman J. Lyme disease-associated glomerulonephritis. *Nephrology Dialysis Transplantation*. 2011;26(9):3054-3056. doi:10.1093/ndt/gfr335. [PubMed] Papineni P, Doherty T, Pickett T, Toth T, Boddana P. Membranous glomerulonephritis secondary to Borrelia burgdorferi infection presenting as nephrotic syndrome. *Clinical Kidney Journal*. 2009;3(1):105-106. doi:10.1093/ndtplus/sfp160. [PubMed] Rawal B, Rovner L, Thakar C, Pollock J. 221: MPGN and Nephrotic Syndrome (NS) Secondary to Lyme Disease (LD). *American Journal of Kidney Diseases*. 2008;51(4):B83. doi:10.1053/j.ajkd.2008.02.231. [http://www.ajkd.org/article/S0272-6386(08)00402-2/abstract]

Lyme hepatitis **	**References** Comstock LE, Thomas DD. Penetration of endothelial cell monolayers by *Borrelia burgdorferi*, *Infect Immun* , 1989, vol. 57 (pg. 1626-8) [PubMed] Goellner MH, Agger WA, Burgess JH, Duray PH. Hepatitis due to recurrent Lyme disease, *Ann Intern Med* , 1988, vol. 108 (pg. 707-8) [PubMed] Schaible UE, Gay S, Museteanu C, et al. . Lyme borreliosis in the severe combined immunodeficiency (*scid*) mouse manifests predominantly in the joint, heart and liver, *Am J Pathol*, 1990, vol. 137 (pg. 811-20) [PubMed] Zaidi SA, Singer C. Gastrointestinal and Hepatic Manifestations of Tickborne Diseases in the United States. *Clin Infect Dis.* 2002:34(9):1206-1212. DOI:https://doi.org/10.1086/339871 [PubMed]
Lyme lymphadeno-pathy is not a separate condition	Błazejewicz-Zawadzińiska M, Brochocka A, Lisińska J, Borowiecki M. [A reprospective analysis of 973 patients with lyme borreliosis in Kuyavian-Pomeranian voivodship in 2000-2005]. [Article in Polish] Przegl Epidemiol. 2012;66(4):581-6. [PubMed] Tunev SS, Hastey CJ, Hodzic E, Feng S, Barthold SW, Baumgarth N. Lymphoadenopathy during lyme borreliosis is caused by spirochete migration-induced specific B cell activation. *PLoS Pathog.* 2011;7(5):e1002066. doi: 10.1371/journal.ppat.1002066. [PubMed] Vukadinov J1, Canak G, Brkić S, Samardzija NM, Aleksić-Dordević M, Turkulov V, Cik-Nad E, Lalosević V. [Clinico-epidemiologic characteristics of Lyme disease treated at the Infectious Disease in Novy Sad 1993-1998]. [Article in Croatian] *Med Pregl.* 2001;54(9-10):470-5. [PubMed]

Lyme myositis	**References** Brtkova J, Jirickova P, Kapla J, Dedic K, Pliskova L. Borrelia arthritis and chronic myositis accompanied by typical chronic dermatitis. *JBR-BTR*. 2008;91(3):88-9. [PubMed] Carvounis PE, Mehta AP, Geist CE. Orbital myositis associated with Borrelia burgdorferi (Lyme disease) infection. *Ophthalmology*. 2004;111(5):1023-8. DOI: 10.1016/j.ophtha.2003.08.032. [PubMed] Holak H, Holak N, Huzarska M, Holak S. Tick inoculation in an eyelid region: report on five cases with one complication of the orbital myositis associated with Lyme borreliosis. *Klin Oczna*. 2006;108(4-6):220-4. [PubMed] Holmgren AR, Matteson EL. Lyme myositis. *Arthritis Rheum*. 2006;54(8):2697-700. [PubMed] Sauer A, Speeg-Schatz C, Hansmann Y. Two cases of orbital myositis as a rare feature of lyme borreliosis. *Case Rep Infect Dis*. 2011;2011:372470. doi: 10.1155/2011/372470. [PubMed] Waton J, Pinault AL, Pouaha J, Truchetet F. [Lyme disease could mimic dermatomyositis]. [Article in French] *Rev Med Interne*. 2007 May;28(5):343-5. [PubMed]
Other conditions	Brooke E. Salzman, MD, Amber Stonehouse, MD and James Studdiford, MD Late Diagnosis of Early Disseminated Lyme Disease: Perplexing Symptoms in a Gardener, J Am Board Fam Med May-June 2008 vol. 21 no. 3 234-236 [PubMed] doi: 10.3122/jabfm.2008.03.070196 Mehrzad R, Bravoco J. Pancytopenia in Lyme disease. *BMJ Case Rep*. 2014;4;2014. pii: bcr2013201079. doi: 10.1136/bcr-2013-201079. [PubMed] Sathiamoorthi S, Smith W. The eye and tick-borne disease in the United States. *Curr Opin Ophthalmol*. 2016 Nov;27(6):530-537. [PubMed]

TABLE 7 Late Lyme Cardiovascular disease

Lyme aortic aneurysm **	References
	Cuisset T, Hamilos M, Vanderheyden M. Coronary aneurysm in Lyme disease: Treatment by covered stent. *International Journal of Cardiology*. 2008;128(2):e72-e73. doi:10.1016/j.ijcard.2007.04.163. [PubMed]
	Gasser R, Watzinger N, Eber B et al. Coronary artery aneurysm in two patients with long-standing Lyme borreliosis. *The Lancet*. 1994;344(8932):1300-1301. doi:10.1016/s0140-6736(94)90789-7. [PubMed]
	Hinterseher I1, Gäbel G, Corvinus F, Lück C, Saeger HD, Bergert H, Tromp G, Kuivaniemi H. Presence of Borrelia burgdorferi sensu lato antibodies in the serum of patients with abdominal aortic aneurysms. Eur J Clin Microbiol Infect Dis. 2012 May;31(5):781-9. doi: 10.1007/s10096-011-1375-y. Epub 2011 Aug 13. [PubMed]
	Watzinger N, Fruhwald F, Schafhalter I et al. [Coronary aneurysm in a 69-year-old patient. Transthoracic echocardiography]. *Ultraschall in der Medizin - European Journal of Ultrasound*. 1995;16(04):200-202. doi:10.1055/s-2007-1003939. [PubMed]
	Xu L1, Heath J, Burke A. Ascending aortitis: a clinicopathological study of 21 cases in a series of 300 aortic repairs. Pathology. 2014 Jun;46(4):296-305. doi: 10.1097/PAT.0000000000000096. [PubMed]
Coronary artery aneurysm	Gasser R, Watzinger N, Eber B, Luha O, Reisinger E, Seinost G, Klein W. Coronary artery aneurysm in two patients with long-standing Lyme borreliosis. Borreliosis Study Group. Lancet. 1994;344:1300-1301. doi: 10.1016/S0140-6736(94)90789-7. [PubMed] [Cross Ref]
	Clinckaert C, Bidgoli S, Verbeet T, Attou R, Gottignies P, Massaut J, Reper P. Peroperative cardiogenic shock suggesting acute coronary syndrome as initial manifestation of Lyme carditis. J Clin Anesth. 2016 Dec;35:430-433. doi: 10.1016/j.jclinane.2016.08.005. Epub 2016 Oct 18. [PubMed]
	Cuisset T, Hamilos M, Vanderheyden M. **Coronary** aneurysm in **Lyme Disease**: treatment by covered stent. Int J Cardiol. 2008 Aug 18;128(2):e72-3. [PubMed]
	Watzinger N, Fruhwald FM, Schafhalter I, Hermann J, Luha O, Zweiker R, Gasser R, Eber B, Klein W. [**Coronary** aneurysm in a 69-year-old patient. Transthoracic echocardiography]. Ultraschall Med. 1995 Aug;16(4):200-2. German. [PubMed]

Late Lyme endocarditis **	**References** Błaut-Jurkowska J, Olszowska M, Kaźnica-Wiatr M, Piotr Podolec P. [Lyme carditis]. [Article in Polish]. *Pol Med J.* 2015;39(230):111-115. [PubMed] Kuchynka P, Palecek T, Havranek S et al. Recent-onset dilated cardiomyopathy associated with Borrelia burgdorferi infection. *Herz.* 2015;40(6):892-897. doi:10.1007/s00059-015-4308-1. [PubMed] Plocarová K. [Inflammatory borrelia - associated dilated cardiomyopathy]. [Article in Czech]. *Vnitr Lek.* 2013;59(12):1107-10. [PubMed]
Lyme carditis **	Avitabile C, Harris M, Chowdhury D. Cardiac Magnetic Resonance Characterizes Myocarditis in a 16-Year-Old Female With Lyme Disease. *World Journal for Pediatric and Congenital Heart Surgery.* 2016;7(3):394-396. doi:10.1177/2150135115593134. [PubMed] Bacino L, Gazzarata M, Siri G, Cordone S, Bellotti P. [Complete atrioventricular block as the first clinical manifestation of a tick bite (Lyme disease)] [in Italian]. *Giornale italiano di cardiologia (2006).* 2011;12(3):214-6. [PubMed] Clinckaert C, Bidgoli S, Verbeet T, et al. Peroperative cardiogenic shock suggesting acute coronary syndrome as initial manifestation of Lyme carditis. *Journal of Clinical Anesthesia.* 2016;35:430-433. doi:10.1016/j.jclinane.2016.08.005. [PubMed] Dernedde S, Piper C, Kühl U, et al. [The Lyme carditis as a rare differential diagnosis to an anterior myocardial infarction] [in German]. *Zeitschrift für Kardiologie.* 2002;91(12):1053-1060. doi:10.1007/s00392-002-0873-4. [PubMed] Guenther F, Bode C, Faber T. [Reversible complete heart block by re-infection with Borrelia burgdorferi with negative IgM-antibodies] [in German]. *Deutsche medizinische Wochenschrift (1946).* 2008;134:23-6. [PubMed] Karadag B, Spieker L, Schwitter J et al. Lyme carditis: restitutio ad integrum documented by cardiac magnetic resonance imaging. *Cardiology in Review.* 2004;12(4):185-187. doi:10.1097/01.crd.0000123841.02777.5d. [PubMed] Kostić T, Momčilović S, Perišić Z et al. Manifestations of Lyme carditis. *International Journal of Cardiology.* 2017;232:24-32. doi:10.1016/j.ijcard.2016.12.169. [PubMed] Kubánek M, Šramko M, Berenová D, et al. Detection of Borrelia burgdorferi sensu lato in endomyocardial biopsy specimens in individuals with recent-onset dilated cardiomyopathy. *European Journal of Heart Failure.* 2012;14(6):588-596. doi:10.1093/eurjhf/hfs027. [PubMed]

Lyme carditis **	References
	Meimoun P, Sayah S, Benali T, et al. [Lyme disease presenting as infarction pain. A case report] [in French]. *Archives des maladies du coeur et des vaisseaux*. 2002;94(12):1419-22. [PubMed] Rostoff P, Konduracka E, Massri E, et al. [Lyme carditis presenting as acute coronary syndrome: A case report] [in Polish]. *Kardiologia polska*. 2008;66(4):420-5. [PubMed] Rudenko N, Golovchenko M, Mokracek A, et al. Detection of Borrelia bissettii in cardiac valve tissue of a patient with Endocarditis and Aortic valve Stenosis in the Czech Republic. *Journal of Clinical Microbiology*. 2008;46(10):3540-3543. doi:10.1128/jcm.01032-08. [PubMed] Sauvant G, Bossart W, Kurrer M, Follath F. [Diagnosis and course of myocarditis: A survey in the medical clinics of Zurich university hospital 1980 to 1998] [in German]. *Schweizerische medizinische Wochenschrift*. 2000;130(36):1265-71. [PubMed] Stanek G, Klein J, Bittner R, Glogar D. Borrelia burgdorferi as an etiologic agent in chronic heart failure? *Scandinavian journal of infectious diseases. Supplementum*. 1991;77:85-7. [PubMed]

TABLE 8 Late NB - neuritis or neuropathy, meningovascular, NB with cerebral infarcts, Lyme parkinsonism, Lyme encephalitis

Symptomatic Late Lyme neuroborreliosis **	References
	Burakgazi AZ. Lyme disease –induced polyradiculopathy mimicking amyotrophic lateral sclerosis. *Inter J of Neuroscience*. 2014;124(11):859-862. doi:10.3109/00207454.2013.879582. [PubMed]
	Christova I, Komitova R. Clinical and epidemiological features of Lyme borreliosis in Bulgaria. *Wien Klin Wochenschr*. 2004;116(1-2):42-6. [PubMed]
	Lawrence C, Lipton RB, Lowy FD, Coyle PK. Seronegative Chronic Relapsing Neuroborreliosis. *Eur Neurol* 1995;35:113-117. [PubMed]
	Marconi RT, Hohenberger S, Jauris-Heipke S, Schulte-Spechtel U, LaVoie CP, Rößler D, Wilske B. Genetic Analysis of Borrelia garinii OspA Serotype 4 Strains Associated with Neuroborreliosis: Evidence for Extensive Genetic Homogeneity. *J Clin Microbiol*. 1999;37(12): 3965-3970. [PubMed Central]
	Nafeev AA, Klimova LV. [Clinical manifestations of neuroborreliosis in the Volga region]. [Article in Russian]. *Ter Arkh*. 2010;82(11):68-70. [PubMed]
Late Lyme neuritis or neuropathy **	Habek M, Mubrin Z, Brinar VV. Avellis syndrome due to borreliosis. *Eur J Neurol*. 2007;14(1):112-4. DOI: 10.1111/j.1468-1331.2006.01528.x. [PubMed]
	Halperin JJ, Little BW, Coyle PK, Dattwyler RJ. Lyme disease: cause of a treatable peripheral neuropathy. *Neurology*. 1987;37(11):1700-6. [PubMed]
	Krim E, Guehl D, Burbaud P, and LaguenyA. Retrobulbar optic neuritis: a complication of Lyme disease? *J Neurol Neurosurg Psychiatry*. 2007;78(12): 1409-1410. doi: 10.1136/jnnp.2006.113761. [PubMed Central]
	Midgard R, Hofstad H. Unusual manifestations of nervous system Borrelia burgdorferi infection. *Arch Neurol*. 1987;44(7):781-3. [PubMed]
	Rothermel H, Hedges TR 3rd, Steere AC. Optic neuropathy in children with Lyme disease. *Pediatrics*. 200;108(2):477-81. [PubMed]
	Träisk F, Lindquist L. Optic nerve involvement in Lyme disease. *Curr Opin Ophthalmol*. 2012;23(6):485-90. doi:10.1097/ICU.0b013e328358b1eb. [PubMed]

Meningovascular & Neuroborreliosis - with cerebral infarcts **	**References** Almoussa M1, Goertzen A1, Fauser B1, Zimmermann CW1. Stroke as an Unusual First Presentation of Lyme Disease. *Case Rep Neurol Med*. 2015;2015:389081. doi: 10.1155/2015/389081. Epub 2015 Dec 16. [PubMed] Back T1, Grünig S, Winter Y, Bodechtel U, Guthke K, Khati D, von Kummer R. Neuroborreliosis-associated cerebral vasculitis: long-term outcome and health-related quality of life. *J Neurol*. 2013 Jun;260(6):1569-75. doi: 10.1007/s00415-013-6831-4. [PubMed] Blažina K, Miletić V, Relja M, Bažadona D. Cerebral sinuvenous thrombosis: a rare complication of Lyme neuroborreliosis. *Wiener klinische Wochenschrift*. 2014;127(1-2):65-67. doi:10.1007/s00508-014-0622-5. [PubMed] Brogan GX, Homan CS, Viccellio P. The enlarging clinical spectrum of Lyme disease: Lyme cerebral vasculitis, a new disease entity. *Ann Emerg Med*. 1990;19:572-6. [PubMed] Defer G, Levy R, Brugieres P, Postic D, Degos JD. Lyme disease presenting as a stroke in the vertebrobasilar territory: MRI. *Neuroradiology*. 1993;35:529-31. [PubMed] Hammers-Berggren S, Grondahl A, Karlsson M, von Arbin M, Carlsson A, Stiernstedt G. Screening for neuroborreliosis in patients with stroke. *Stroke*. 1993;24:1393-6. [PubMed] Hanny PE, Hauselmann HJ. [Lyme disease from the neurologist's viewpoint]. [in German]. *Schweiz Med Wochenschr*. 1987;117:901-15. [PubMed] Heinrich A, Khaw AV, Ahrens N, Kirsch M, Dressel A. Cerebral vasculitis as the only manifestation of Borrelia burgdorferi infection in a 17-year-old patient with basal ganglia infarction. *Eur Neurol*. 2003;50:109-12. [PubMed] Keil R, Baron R, Kaiser R, Deuschl G. [Vasculitis course of neuroborreliosis with thalamic infarct]. [in German]. *Nervenarzt*. 1997;68:339-41. [PubMed] Klingebiel R, Benndorf G, Schmitt M, von Moers A, Lehmann R. Large cerebral vessel occlusive disease in Lyme neuroborreliosis. *Neuropediatrics*. 2002;33:37-40. [PubMed] Kraemer M, Berlit P. Systemic, secondary and infectious causes for cerebral vasculitis: clinical experience with 16 new European cases. *Rheumatology International*. 2009;30(11):1471-1476. doi:10.1007/s00296-009-1172-4. [PubMed]

Meningovascular & Neuroborreliosis - with cerebral infarcts **	**References** Kuntzer T, Bogousslavsky J, Miklossy J, Steck AJ, Janzer R, Regli F. Borrelia rhombencephalomyelopathy. *Arch Neurol*. 1991;48:832-6. [PubMed] Kurian M, Pereira VM, Vargas MI, Fluss J. Stroke-like Phenomena Revealing Multifocal Cerebral Vasculitis in Pediatric Lyme Neuroborreliosis. *J Child Neurol*. 2015 Aug;30(9):1226-9. doi: 10.1177/0883073814552104. [PubMed] Laroche C, Lienhardt A, Boulesteix J. [Ischemic stroke caused by neuroborreliosis]. [in French]. *Arch Pediatr*. 1999;6(12):1302-5. [PubMed] Lebas A, Toulgoat F, Saliou G, Husson B, Tardieu M. Stroke Due to Lyme Neuroborreliosis: Changes in Vessel Wall Contrast Enhancement. *J Neuroimag*. 2012;22(12):210-2. [PubMed] May EF, Jabbari B. Stroke in neuroborreliosis. *Stroke*. 1990;21:1232-5. [PubMed] Midgard R, Hofstad H. Unusual manifestations of nervous system Borrelia burgdorferi infection. *Arch Neurol*. 1987;44:781-3. [PubMed] Miklossy J, Kuntzer T, Bogousslavsky J, Regli F, Janzer RC. Meningovascular form of neuroborreliosis: similarities between neuropathological findings in a case of Lyme disease and those occurring in tertiary neurosyphilis. *Acta Neuropathol*. 1990;80:568-72. [PubMed] Miklossy J. Biology and neuropathology of dementia in syphilis and Lyme disease. *Handb Clin Neurol*. 2008;89:825-44. [PubMed] Olsson JE, Zbornikova V. Neuroborreliosis simulating a progressive stroke. *Acta Neurol Scand*. 1990;81:471-4. [PubMed] Reik L., Jr Stroke due to Lyme disease. *Neurology*. 1993;43:2705-7. [PubMed] Rey V, Du Pasquier R, Muehl A, Peter O, Michel P. [Multiple ischemic strokes due to Borrelia garinii meningovasculitis]. [in French]. *Rev Neurol (Paris)* 2010;166:931-4. [PubMed] Romi F, Krakenes J, Aarli JA, Tysnes OB. Neuroborreliosis with vasculitis causing stroke-like manifestations. *Eur Neurol*. 2004;51:49-50. [PubMed]

Meningovascular & Neuroborreliosis - with cerebral infarcts **	**References** Schmiedel J, Gahn G, von Kummer R, Reichmann H. Cerebral vasculitis with multiple infarcts caused by lyme disease. *Cerebrovasc Dis.* 2004;17:79-81. [PubMed] Schmitt AB, Kuker W, Nacimiento W. [Neuroborreliosis with extensive cerebral vasculitis and multiple cerebral infarcts]. [in German]. *Nervenarzt.* 1999;70:167-71. [PubMed] Shadick NA, Phillips CB, Logigian EL, et al. The long-term clinical outcomes of Lyme disease. A population-based retrospective cohort study. *Ann Intern Med.* 1994;121:560-7. [PubMed] Sparsa L, Blanc F, Lauer V, Cretin B, Marescaux C, Wolff V. Recurrent ischemic strokes revealing Lyme meningovascularitis. *Rev Neurol (Paris)* 2009;165:273-7. [PubMed] Topakian R, Stieglbauer K, Aichner FT. Unexplained cerebral vasculitis and stroke: keep Lyme neuroborreliosis in mind. *Lancet Neurol.* 2007;6:756-7. [PubMed] Uldry PA, Regli F, Bogousslavsky J. Cerebral angiopathy and recurrent strokes following Borrelia burgdorferi infection. *J Neurol Neurosurg Psychiat.* 1987;50:1703-4. [PubMed Central] Van Snick S, Duprez TP, Kabamba B, Van De Wyngaert FA, Sindic CJ. Acute ischaemic pontine stroke revealing lyme neuroborreliosis in a young adult. *Acta Neurol Belg.* 2008;108:103-6. [PubMed] Veenendaal-Hilbers JA, Perquin WV, Hoogland PH, Doornbos L. Basal meningovasculitis and occlusion of the basilar artery in two cases of Borrelia burgdorferi infection. *Neurology.* 1988;38:1317-9. [PubMed] Wittwer B, Pelletier S, Ducrocq X, Maillard L, Mione G, Richard S. Cerebrovascular Events in Lyme Neuroborreliosis. *J Stroke Cerebrovasc Dis.* 2015 Jul;24(7):1671-8. doi: 10.1016/j.jstrokecerebrovasdis.2015.03.056. [PubMed] Zajkowska J, Garkowski A, Moniuszko A et al. Vasculitis and stroke due to Lyme neuroborreliosis - a review. *Infectious Diseases.* 2014;47(1):1-6. doi:10.3109/00365548.2014.961544. [PubMed] Zhang Y, Lafontant G, Bonner FJ., Jr Lyme neuroborreliosis mimics stroke: a case report. *Arch phys Med Rehab.* 2000;81:519-21. [PubMed]

Intracranial aneurysm **	**References** Oksi J, Kalimo H, Marttila RJ, Marjamäki M, Sonninen P, Nikoskelainen J, Viljanen MK. Intracranial aneurysms in three patients with disseminated Lyme borreliosis: cause or chance association? J Neurol Neurosurg Psychiatry. 1998;64:636-642. doi: 10.1136/jnnp.64.5.636. [PMC free article] [PubMed] Polet JD, Weinstein HC. Lyme borreliosis and intracranial aneurysm. J Neurol Neurosurg Psychiatry. 1999;66:806-807. doi: 10.1136/jnnp.66.6.806a. [PMC free article] [PubMed]
Lyme Parkinsonism	Cassarino DS, Quezado MM, Ghatak NR, Duray PH. Lyme-associated parkinsonism: a neuropathologic case study and review of the literature. *Arch Pathol Lab Med.* 2003;127(9):1204-6. [PubMed] Scholz SW, Bras J. Genetics Underlying Atypical Parkinsonism and Related Neurodegenerative Disorders. Jellinger KA, ed. *International Journal of Molecular Sciences.* 2015;16(10):24629-24655. doi:10.3390/ijms161024629 [PubMed]
Late Lyme encephalitis **	Rocha R, Lisboa L, Neves J, García López M, Santos E, Ribeiro A. Neuroborreliosis Presenting as Acute Disseminated Encephalomyelitis. *Pediatric Emergency Care.* 2012;28(12):1374-1376. doi:10.1097/pec.0b013e318276c51d. [PubMed] Verma V, Roman MShah D, Zaretskaya M, Yassin MH. A case of chronic progressive lyme encephalitis as a manifestation of late lyme neuroborreliosis. Infect Dis Rep. 2014 Dec 11;6(4):5496. doi: 10.4081/idr.2014.5496. eCollection 2014 [PubMed]
Symptomatic Lyme neuroborreliosis, unspecified **	Miklossy J. Chronic or late lyme neuroborreliosis: analysis of evidence compared to chronic or late neurosyphilis. Open Neurol J. 2012;6:146-57. doi: 10.2174/1874205X01206010146. Epub 2012 Dec 28. [PubMed] Miklossy J (2015) Historic evidence to support a causal relationship between spirochetal infections and Alzheimer's disease. Front Aging Neurosci 7, 46. [PMC free article] [PubMed] Yoshinari NH, de Barros PJ, Bonoldi VL, Ishikawa M, Battesti DM, Pirana S, da Fonseca AH, Schumaker TT. [Outline of Lyme borreliosis in Brazil]. [in Portuguese]. *Rev Hosp Clin Fac Med Sao Paulo.* 1997;52(2):111-7. [PubMed]

TABLE 9 neuroborreliosis - Late Lyme meningoencephalitis or meningomyeloencephalitis

Late Lyme meningo-encephalitis or meningomyelo encephalitis **	References
	Ackermann R, Gollmer E, Rehse-Küpper B. [Progressive Borrelia encephalomyelitis. Chronic manifestation of erythema chronicum migrans disease of the nervous system]. [in German]. *DMW - Deutsche Medizinische Wochenschrift*. 1985;110(26):1039-1042. doi:10.1055/s-2008-1068956. [PubMed] Bensch J, Olcen P, Hagberg L. Destructive chronic borrelia meningoencephalitis in a child untreated for 15 years. *Scand J Infect Dis*. 1987;19:697-700. [PubMed] Bertrand E, Szpak GM, Pilkowska E, et al. Central nervous system infection caused by Borrelia burgdorferi. Clinico-pathological correlation of three post-mortem cases. *Folia neuropathologica*. 1999;37:43-51. [PubMed] Bogsrud T, Odegaard B. [Tick-borne borreliosis. A case of chronic meningoencephalitis caused by Borrelia burgdorferi]. [in Norwegian]. *Tidsskr Nor Laegeforen*. 1987;107(1):25-7, 49. [PubMed] Cassarino DS, Quezado MM, Ghatak NR, Duray PH. Lyme-associated parkinsonism: a neuropathologic case study and review of the literature. *Arch Pathol Lab Med*. 2003;127:1204-6. [PubMed] Czyrny M, Jura E, Seniow J, Baranska M, Wilske B, Czlonkowska A. [Severe meningoencephalitis in Borrelia burgdorferi infection]. [in Polish]. *Neurol Neurochir Pol*. 1998;32:387-93. [PubMed] De Cauwer H, Declerck S, De Smet J, et al. Motor neuron disease features in a patient with neuroborreliosis and a cervical anterior horn lesion. *Acta clinica Belgica*. 2009;64:225-7. [PubMed] Diringer MN, Halperin JJ, Dattwyler RJ. Lyme meningoencephalitis: report of a severe, penicillin-resistant case. *Arthritis Rheum*. 1987;30:705-8. [PubMed] Drouet A, Meyer X, Guilloton L, et al. [Acute severe leukoencephalitis with posterior lesions due to Borrelia burgdorferi infection]. [in French]. *Presse Med*. 2003;32:1607-9. [PubMed] Duray PH, Steere AC. Clinical pathologic correlations of Lyme disease by stage. *Ann N Y Acad Sci*. 1988;539:65-79. [PubMed]

Late Lyme meningo-encephalitis or meningomyelo-encephalitis **	**References** Duray PH, Steere AC. The spectrum of organ and systems pathology in human Lyme disease. *Zentralbl Bakteriol Mikrobiol Hyg A*. 1986;263:169-78. [PubMed] Duray PH. Histopathology of clinical phases of human Lyme disease. *Rheum Dis Clin North Am*. 1989;15:691-710. [PubMed] Duray PH. The surgical pathology of human Lyme disease. An enlarging picture. *Am J Surg Pathol*. 1987;11(Suppl 1):47-60. [PubMed] Fénelon G, Chaine P, Lèche J, Guillard A. [Isolated meningoencephalitis in Lyme disease]. [in French]. *Ann Med Interne (Paris)*. 1987;138(2):149-50. [PubMed] Ferroir J, Reignier A, Nicolle M, Guillard A. [Meningoradiculoencephalitis in Lyme disease. A case with major regressive mental disorders], [in French]. *Presse Med*. 1988;17(14):697. [PubMed] Kacinski M, Zajac A, Skowronek-Bala B, Kroczka S, Gergont A, Kubik A. CNS Lyme disease manifestation in children. *Przeglad lekarski*. 2007;64(Suppl 3):38-40. [PubMed] Kawano Y, Shigeto H, Shiraishi Y, Ohyagi Y, Kira J. Case of Borrelia brainstem encephalitis presenting with severe dysphagia. *Clin Neurol*. 2010;50:265-7. [PubMed] Nadelman RB, Nowakowski J, Forseter G, et al. The clinical spectrum of early Lyme borreliosis in patients with culture-confirmed erythema migrans. Am J Med. 1996;100:502-8. [PubMed] Neumarker KJ, Dudeck U, Plaza P. [Borrelia encephalitis and catatonia in adolescence]. [in German]. *Nervenarzt*. 1989;60:115-9. [PubMed] Oksi J, Kalimo H, Marttila RJ, et al. Inflammatory brain changes in Lyme borreliosis. A report on three patients and review of literature. *Brain*. 1996;119(Pt 6):2143-54. [PubMed] Oksi J, Viljanen MK, Kalimo H, et al. Fatal encephalitis caused by concomitant infection with tick-borne encephalitis virus and Borrelia burgdorferi. *Clinical infectious diseases: an official publication of the Infectious. Dis Soc Am*. 1993;16:392-6. [PubMed]

Late Lyme meningo-encephalitis or meningomy-eloencephalitis **	References
	Omasits M, Seiser A, Brainin M. [Recurrent and relapsing course of borreliosis of the nervous system]. [in German]. *Wien Klin Wochenschr*. 1990;102:4-12. [PubMed]
	Oschmann P, Dorndorf W, Hornig C, Schafer C, Wellensiek HJ, Pflughaupt KW. Stages and syndromes of neuroborreliosis. *J Neurol*. 1998;245:262-72. [PubMed]
	Pachner AR, Duray P, Steere AC. Central nervous system manifestations of Lyme disease. *Arch Neurol*. 1989;46:790-5. [PubMed]
	Pennekamp A, Jaques M. [Chronic neuroborreliosis with gait ataxia and cognitive disorders]. [in German]. *Praxis (Bern 1994)*. 1997;86(20):867-9. [PubMed]
	Pfefferkorn T, Feddersen B, Schulte-Altedorneburg G, Linn J, Pfister HW. Tick-borne encephalitis with polyradiculitis documented by MRI. *Neurology*. 2007;68:1232-3. [PubMed]
	Ponz E, Graus F, Alvarez R, Sarmiento X, Vidal J, Grau JM. [Meningoencephalomyelitis caused by Borrelia burgdorferi: a case without epidemiologic history or chronic migratory erythema]. [in Spanish]. *Med Clin (Barc)*. 1989;93:218-20. [PubMed]
	Reik L Jr, Burgdorfer W, Donaldson JO. Neurologic abnormalities in Lyme disease without erythema chronicum migrans. *Am J Med*. 1986;81:73-8. [PubMed]
	Shadick NA, Phillips CB, Logigian EL, et al. The long-term clinical outcomes of Lyme disease. A population-based retrospective cohort study. *Ann Intern Med*. 1994;121:560-7. [PubMed]
	Weder B, Wiedersheim P, Matter L, Steck A, Otto F. Chronic progressive neurological involvement in Borrelia burgdorferi infection. *J Neurol*. 1987;234:40-3. [PubMed]

TABLE 10 Late atrophic form of Lyme meningoencephalitis with dementia &
subacute presenile dementia & Neuropsychiatric manifestations

Atrophic form of Lyme meningo-encephalitis with dementia & subacute presenile dementia **	References
	Aasly J, Nilsen G. Cerebral atrophy in Lyme disease. *Neuroradiology*. 1990;32:252. [PubMed]
	Allen HB, Morales D. Alzheimers disease: A novel hypothesis integrating spirochetes, biofilm, and the immune system. *Journal of Neuroinfectious Diseases*. 2016;07(01). doi:10.4172/2314-7326.1000200. [https://www.researchgate.net/publication/294089000_Alzheimer's_Disease_A_Novel_Hypothesis_Integrating_Spirochetes_Biofilm_and_the_Immune_System]
	Almeida OP, Lautenschlager NT. Dementia associated with infectious diseases. *International Psychogeriatrics*. 2005;17(S1):S65. doi:10.1017/s104161020500195x. [PubMed]
	Bu X, Yao X, Jiao S et al. A study on the association between infectious burden and Alzheimer's disease. *European Journal of Neurology*. 2014;22(12):1519-1525. doi:10.1111/ene.12477. [PubMed]
	Dupuis MJ. Multiple neurologic manifestations of Borrelia burgdorferi infection. *Rev Neurol*. 1988;144:765-75. [PubMed]
	Duray PH. The surgical pathology of human Lyme disease. An enlarging picture. *Am J Surg Pathol*. 1987;11(Suppl 1):47-60. [PubMed]
	Itzhaki R, Lathe R, Balin B et al. Microbes and Alzheimer's Disease. *Journal of Alzheimer's Disease*. 2016;51(4):979-984. doi:10.3233/jad-160152. [PubMed]
	Juchnowicz D, Rudnik I, Czernikiewicz A, Zajkowska J, Pancewicz SA. [Mental disorders in the course of lyme borreliosis and tick borne encephalitis] [in Polish]. *Przeglad epidemiologiczny*. 2002;56:37-50. [PubMed]
	Koc F, Bozdemir H, Pekoz T, Aksu H, Ozcan S, Kurdak H. Lyme disease presenting as subacute transverse myelitis. *Acta Neurol Belg*. 2009;109(4):326-9. [PubMed]
	MacDonald A, Miranda J. Concurrent neocortical borreliosis and Alzheimer's disease. *Human Pathology*. 1987;18(7):759-761. doi:10.1016/s0046-8177(87)80252-6. [PubMed]
	MacDonald AB. Borrelia in the brains of patients dying with dementia. *JAMA*. 1986;256:2195-6. [PubMed]

Atrophic form of Lyme meningo-encephalitis with dementia & subacute presenile dementia **	**References** Mawanda F, Wallace R. Can infections cause Alzheimer's disease? *Epidemiologic Reviews*. 2013;35(1):161-180. doi:10.1093/epirev/mxs007. [PubMed] Miklossy J, Gern L, Darekar P, Janzer RC, Van der Loos H. Senile plaques, neurofibrillary tangles and neuropil threads contain DNA? *Journal of Spirochetal and Tick Borne-Diseases*. 1995;2:1-5. Miklossy J, Kasas S, Janzer RC, Ardizzoni F, Van der Loos H. Further ultrastructural evidence that spirochaetes may play a role in the aetiology of Alzheimer's disease. *Neuroreport*. 1994;5:1201-4. [PubMed] Miklossy J, Kasas S, Zurn A, McCall S, Yu S, McGeer P. Persisting atypical and cystic forms of Borrelia burgdorferi and local inflammation in Lyme neuroborreliosis. *Journal of Neuroinflammation*. 2008;5(1):40. doi:10.1186/1742-2094-5-40. [PubMed] Miklossy J, Khalili K, Gern L, et al. Borrelia burgdorferi persists in the brain in chronic Lyme neuroborreliosis and may be associated with Alzheimer disease. *Journal of Alzheimer's Disease*. 2004;6(6):639-649. [PubMed] Miklossy J, Kis A, Radenovic A, et al. Beta-amyloid deposition and Alzheimer's type changes induced by Borrelia spirochetes. *Neurobiology of Aging*. 2006;27(2):228-236. doi:10.1016/j.neurobiolaging.2005.01.018. [PubMed] Miklossy J. Alzheimer's disease - a neurospirochetosis. Analysis of the evidence following Koch's and hill's criteria. *Journal of Neuroinflammation*. 2011;8(1):90. doi:10.1186/1742-2094-8-90. [PMC free article] [PubMed] Miklossy J. Alzheimer's disease--a spirochetosis? *Neuroreport*. 1993;4:841-8. [PubMed] Miklossy J. Bacterial Amyloid and DNA are Important Constituents of Senile Plaques: Further Evidence of the Spirochetal and Biofilm Nature of Senile Plaques. *Journal of Alzheimer's Disease*. 2016;53(4):1459-1473. doi:10.3233/jad-160451. [PubMed]

Atrophic form of Lyme meningo-encephalitis with dementia & subacute presenile dementia **	**References** Miklossy J. Chronic inflammation and amyloidogenesis in Alzheimer's disease -- role of Spirochetes. *Journal of Alzheimer's disease : JAD.* 2008;13(4):381–91. [PubMed] Miklossy J. Emerging roles of pathogens in Alzheimer disease. *Expert Reviews in Molecular Medicine.* 2011;13. doi:10.1017/s1462399411002006. [PubMed] Miklossy J. Historic evidence to support a causal relationship between spirochetal infections and Alzheimer's disease. *Frontiers in Aging Neuroscience.* 2015;7. doi:10.3389/fnagi.2015.00046. [PubMed Central] Miklossy J: The spirochetal etiology of Alzheimer's disease: A putative therapeutic approach. In Alzheimer Disease: Therapeutic Strategies. Proceedings of the Third International Springfield Alzheimer Symposium. Edited by: Giacobini E, Becker R. Birkhauser Boston Inc.; 1994:, Part I: 41-48. Pennekamp A, Jaques M. [Chronic neuroborreliosis with gait ataxia and cognitive disorders] [in German]. *Praxis.* 1997;86(20):867–9. https://www.ncbi.nlm.nih.gov/pubmed/9312817. Accessed February 27, 2017. [PubMed] Reik L Jr, Burgdorfer W, Donaldson JO. Neurologic abnormalities in Lyme disease without erythema chronicum migrans. *Am J Med.* 1986;81:73-8. [PubMed] Schaeffer S, Le Doze F, De la Sayette V, Bertran F, Viader F. Dementia in Lyme disease. *Presse Med.* 1994;23:861. [PubMed] Tarasów E, Ustymowicz A, Zajkowska J, Hermanowska-Szpakowicz T. [Neuroborreliosis: CT and MRI findings in 14 cases. Preliminary communication] [in Polish]. *Neurologia i neurochirurgia polska.* 2002;35(5):803–13. [PubMed] Waniek C, Prohovnik I, Kaufman MA, Dwork AJ. Rapidly progressive frontal-type dementia associated with Lyme disease. *J Neuropsychiatry Clin Neurosci.* 1995;7:345-7. [PubMed]

Neuropsychiatric manifestations	References
	Fallon B, Kochevar J, Gaito A, Nields J. The underdiagnosis of neuropsychiatric lyme disease in children and adults. *Psychiatric Clinics of North America*. 1998;21(3):693-703. doi:10.1016/s0193-953x(05)70032-0. [PubMed]
	Fallon BA, Nields JA. Lyme disease: a neuropsychiatric illness. *The Am J Psychiatr*. 1994;151:1571-83. [PubMed]
	Fallon B, Nields J, Parsons B, Liebowitz M, Klein D. Psychiatric manifestations of Lyme borreliosis. *J Clin Psychiatry*. 1993;54(7):263-8. [Europe PMC] [PubMed]
	Tager FA, Fallon BA, Keilp J, Rissenberg M, Jones CR, Liebowitz MR. A controlled study of cognitive deficits in children with chronic Lyme disease. *J Neuropsychiatry Clin Neurosci.* 2001;13(4):500-7. [PubMed]

TABLE 11 Late Lyme Bone & Joint & Musculoskeletal

Late Lyme borreliosis of bone and joint	References
	Deanehan JK, Kimia AA, Tan Tanny SP, et al. Distinguishing Lyme from septic knee monoarthritis in Lyme disease-endemic areas. *Pediatrics*. 2013;131(3):e695-701. doi:10.1542/peds.2012-2531. [PubMed]
	Jones KL, McHugh GA, Glickstein LJ, Steere AC. Analysis of Borrelia burgdorferi genotypes in patients with Lyme arthritis: High frequency of ribosomal RNA intergenic spacer type 1 strains in antibiotic-refractory arthritis. *Arthritis Rheum*. 2009;60(7):2174-2182. doi:10.1002/art.24812. [PubMed]
	Lesnicar G, Zerdoner D. Temporomandibular joint involvement caused by Borrelia Burgdorferi. *J Cranio-Maxillo-fac Surg Off Publ Eur Assoc Cranio-Maxillo-fac Surg*. 2007;35(8):397-400. doi:10.1016/j.jcms.2007.06.003. [PubMed]
	Pañczuk A, Tokarska-Rodak M, Kozioł-Montewka M, Plewik D. The incidence of Borrelia burgdorferi, Anaplasma phagocytophilum and Babesia microti coinfections among foresters and farmers in eastern Poland. *J Vector Borne Dis*. 2016;53(4):348-354. [PubMed]
	Renaud I, Cachin C, Gerster J-C. Good outcomes of Lyme arthritis in 24 patients in an endemic area of Switzerland. *Jt Bone Spine Rev Rhum*. 2004;71(1):39-43. doi:10.1016/S1297-319X(03)00160-X. [PubMed]
	Schmid G. Epidemiology and Clinical Similarities of Human Spirochetal Diseases. *Clinical Infectious Diseases*. 1989;11(Supplement 6):S1460-S1469. doi: 10.1093/clinids/11.supplement_6.s1460. [PubMed]
	Yoshinari NH, de Barros PJ, Bonoldi VL, Ishikawa M, Battesti DM, Pirana S, da Fonseca AH, Schumaker TT. [Outline of Lyme borreliosis in Brazil]. [in Portuguese]. *Rev Hosp Clin Fac Med Sao Paulo*. 1997;52(2):111-7. [PubMed]
Late Lyme borreliosis of other musculo-skeletal tissue	Lipsker D, Hansmann Y, Limbach F, Clerc C, Tranchant C, Grunenberger F, Caro-Sampara F, Attali P, Frey M, Kubina M, Piémont Y, Sibilia J, Jaulhac B; Disease expression of Lyme borreliosis in northeastern France. *Eur J Clin Microbiol Infect Dis*. 2001;20(4):225-30. [PubMed]
	Wendling D, Sevrin P, Bouchaud-Chabot A, et al. Parsonage-Turner syndrome revealing Lyme borreliosis. *Jt Bone Spine Rev Rhum*. 2009;76(2):202-204. doi:10.1016/j.jbspin.2008.07.013. [PubMed]

TABLE 12 Late – oculopathy & liver & kidney & respiratory

Late Lyme oculopathy	References
	Drenckhahn A, Spors B, Knierim E. Acute isolated partial oculomotor nerve palsy due to Lyme neuroborreliosis in a 5 year old girl. *European Journal of Paediatric Neurology*. 2016;20(6):977-979. doi:10.1016/j.ejpn.2016.05.022. [PubMed] Karma A, Seppälä I, Mikkilä H, Kaakkola S, Viljanen M, Tarkkanen A. Diagnosis and clinical characteristics of ocular Lyme borreliosis. *Am J Ophthalmol*. 1995;119(2):127-135. [PubMed] Golubić D, Vinković T, Turk D, Hranilović J, Slugan I. [Ocular manifestations of Lyme borreliosis in northwest Croatia]. [in Croatian]. *Lijec Vjesn*. 2004;126(5-6):124-128. [PubMed] Mikkilä HO, Seppälä IJ, Viljanen MK, Peltomaa MP, Karma A. The expanding clinical spectrum of ocular lyme borreliosis. *Ophthalmology*. 2000;107(3):581-587. [PubMed]
Late Lyme disease of liver and other viscera **	Krause PJ, Telford SR, Spielman A, et al. Concurrent Lyme disease and babesiosis. Evidence for increased severity and duration of illness. *JAMA*. 1996;275(21):1657-1660. [PubMed] Muslmani M, Gilson M, Sudre A, Juvin R, Gaudin P. [Lyme disease with hepatitis and corticosteroids: a case report]. [in French]. *Rev Med Interne*. 2012;33(6):339-342. doi:10.1016/j.revmed.2012.01.016. [PubMed]

Late Lyme disease of kidney & ureter **	**References** Finnian R. Mc Causland, Sophie Niedermaier, Vanesa Bijol, Helmut G. Rennke, Mary E. Choi, John P. Forman; Lyme disease-associated glomerulonephritis. *Nephrol Dial Transplant* 2011; 26 (9): 3054-3056. doi: 10.1093/ndt/gfr335 [PubMed] Florens N, Lemoine S, Guebre-Egziabher F, et al. Chronic Lyme borreliosis associated with minimal change glomerular disease: a case report. *BMC Nephrol*. 2017;18(1). doi:10.1186/s12882-017-0462-4. [PubMed] Kelly B, Finnegan P, Cormican M, et al. . Lyme disease and glomerulonephritis, *Ir Med J*, 1999, vol. 92 pg. 372 [PubMed] Papineni P, Doherty T, Pickett T, et al. . Membranous glomerulonephritis secondary to *Borrelia burgdorferi* infection presenting as nephrotic syndrome, *NDT Plus*, 2010, vol. 3 (pg. 105-106) [PubMed] Google ScholarPubMed Rawal B, Rovner L, Thakar C, et al. MPGN and nephrotic syndrome secondary to Lyme disease, *Am J Kidney Dis (abstract)*, 2008, vol. 51 pg. B83 Google ScholarCrossRef
Late Lyme disease of Bronchus & lung **	Faul JL, Ruoss S, Doye RL. Diaphgramatic paralysis due to Lyme disease. Eur Respir J. 1999;13:700-702. doi: 10.1183/09031936.99.13370099. [PubMed] [Cross Ref] Nguyen H, Le C, Nguyen H. Acute lyme infection presenting with amyopathic dermatomyositis and rapidly fatal interstitial pulmonary fibrosis: a case report. *J Med Case Reports*. 2010;4(1). doi:10.1186/1752-1947-4-187. [PubMed] Silva MT, Sophar M, Howard RS. Neuroborreliosis as a cause of respiratory failure. J Neurol. 1992;242:604-607. doi: 10.1007/BF00868815. [PubMed] [Cross Ref]

TABLE 13 Latent Lyme disease, unspecified

Latent Lyme disease, unspecified	References
	Coyle PK1, Dattwyler R. Spirochetal infection of the central nervous system. Infect Dis Clin North Am. 1990 Dec;4(4):731-46. PMID: 2277196 [PubMed] Gylfe A, Wahlgren M, Fahlén L, Bergström S. Activation of latent Lyme borreliosis concurrent with a herpes simplex virus type 1 infection. Scand J Infect Dis. 2002;34(12):922-4. PMID:12587627 [PubMed] Lesniak OM, Belikov ES. [The classification of Lyme borreliosis (Lyme disease)]. Ter Arkh. 1995;67(11):49-51. PMID: 8571252 [PubMed] Miklossy J, Kasas S, Zurn AD, McCall S, Yu S, McGeer PL. Persisting atypical and cystic forms of Borrelia burgdorferi and local inflammation in Lyme neuroborreliosis. *J Neuroinflammation*. 2008;5(1):40. doi:10.1186/1742-2094-5-40. [PubMed] Nafeev AA, Klimova LV. [Clinical manifestations of neuroborreliosis in the Volga region]. Ter Arkh. 2010;82(11):68-70. [Article in Russian] [PubMed] Pachner AR. Spirochetal diseases of the CNS. *Neurol Clin*. 1986;4(1):207-222. [PubMed] Pfister HW, Preac-Mursic V, Wilske B, Einhäupl KM, Weinberger K.Latent Lyme neuroborreliosis: presence of Borrelia burgdorferi in the cerebrospinal fluid without concurrent inflammatory signs. Neurology. 1989 Aug;39(8):1118-20. PMID: 2668788 [PubMed] Schmid GP. Epidemiology and clinical similarities of human spirochetal diseases. Rev Infect Dis. 1989;11 Suppl 6:S1460-9. [PubMed] Yoshinari NH, de Barros PJ, Bonoldi VL, Ishikawa M, Battesti DM, Pirana S, da Fonseca AH, Schumaker TT. [Outline of Lyme borreliosis in Brazil]. Rev Hosp Clin Fac Med Sao Paulo. 1997;52(2):111-7. [Article in Portuguese] [PubMed]

VIII. Conclusions

The ICD11 revisions process wisely invites and includes stakeholder engagement which is critical to advancing science that is patient-centered, rational and humane. To date, however, the voices of those living with complicated cases of Lyme borreliosis and relapsing fever borreliosis, and those who treat or are concerned with such patients, have been largely excluded from this consideration. Their engagement has been limited to sending suggestions to a digital portal that has no venue for dialogue or respectful exchange.

This is in striking contrast to stakeholder interaction representing the other diseases WHO has characterized as consequential; such groups have been invited to collaborate with WHO in numerous exchanges.[66]

In addition, there has been little transparency regarding the scientific basis upon which the codes for Lyme and relapsing fever borreliosis are determined – there is no list of the studies informing the borreliosis code revisions readily available to the public.

Peer-reviewed and published scientific and medical studies supporting persistent Lyme infection and symptoms, expert scientific and medical witnesses, patient testimonials, and the high incidence of coinfections and complications from other tick-borne illnesses are officially on government record in many WHO member countries. These include Austria, Australia, Baltic State of Belarus, Belgium, Brazil, Canada, Croatia, the Czech Republic, Denmark, Estonia, France, Finland, Germany, Greece, Iceland, Ireland, Italy, Latvia, Lithuania, Luxembourg, Moldova, the Netherlands, New Zealand, Norway, People's Republic of China, Poland, Kyrgyzstan, Russia, Senegal, Scotland, Slovak Republic, Slovenia, Spain, Switzerland, Sweden, Ukraine, United Kingdom and USA.

There has been a proliferation of laws passed to protect this neglected patient group and those health practitioners who provide their care and educate the public regarding the dangers of this epidemic.

Many of these countries now have nationally and internationally recognized government officials and elected representatives championing treatment options for complicated and persistent cases of Lyme disease. To date, perhaps through oversight, these government officials from WHO member states have not been invited to participate in the revisions of the borreliosis codes.

A considerable body of scientific evidence relating to the acute, subacute, persistent and late manifestations of borreliosis has been amassed over the past four decades. The diseases caused by *Borrelia* genospecies cause illness of high-incidence and significant morbidity. Some pathogenic strains belonging to the *B. burgdorferi* sl complex have a worldwide distribution, yet they are rarely tested for or considered in diagnoses.[67]

The stated recommendations for the updating of the borreliosis codes will have a broad positive impact on multiple fronts. The recommended revisions of the ICD11 codes for LB will:

- Enable more complete and accurate tracking and reporting of the illness
- This modernization will help epidemiologists better understand the disease and governments to better assess the need for funding of research
- Improve data which will in turn increase accuracy of the statistical modeling used for anticipating human health vulnerability with regards to climate change
- Assist physicians to more accurately and comprehensively report the medical status of their patients providing for the proper recognition, diagnosis and treatment of these illnesses
- Advance our understanding of these illnesses
- Support early, accurate diagnosis and treatment leading to recovery from this complex and debilitating disease
- Help patients with Lyme borreliosis and relapsing fever borreliosis will receive wider recognition, validation and commensurate support from health care, insurance, educational, employment and governmental institutions
- Lighten the epidemic's burdens affecting millions around the globe and support the functional independence and well-being of youthful potential and those skilled and able to contribute to societies.

In closing, there are no medical, scientific, economic or other rationale to continue with the current codes and every reason to revise the codes. It is time for WHO to engage with the global borreliosis stakeholder community who recognize the wide-ranging manifestations experienced by borreliosis patients and take leadership to end this epoch of unnecessary suffering and discrimination against those living with complicated and persistent forms of borreliosis disease.

Endnotes

---

[1] Some references from WHO publications regarding Lyme borreliosis follow:
www.who.int/water_sanitation_health/resources/vector262to287.pdf
Vector control - World Health Organization 1995. Public health importance CHAPTER 4 • BEDBUGS, FLEAS, LICE, TICKS AND MITES Page 268 - Tick-borne relapsing fever, Page 269 - Lyme disease
http://www.who.int/globalchange/publications/climchange.pdf
Climate change and human health RISKS AND RESPONSES - WHO 2003 (IPCC contribution) CHAPTER 6 - Climate change and infectious diseases J. A. Patz, A. K. Githeko, J. P. McCarty, S. Hussein, U. Confalonieri, N. de Wet Page 125 - BOX 6.2 Ecological influences and Lyme disease
www.euro.who.int/ data/assets/pdf_file/0008/98765/e82481.pdf
THE VECTOR-BORNE HUMAN INFECTIONS OF EUROPE - THEIR DISTRIBUTION AND BURDEN ON PUBLIC HEALTH
http://www.euro.who.int/_____data/assets/pdf_file/0006/96819/E89522.pdf
Lyme borreliosis in Europe: influences of climate and climate change, epidemiology, ecology and adaptation measures by Elisabet Lindgren, Thomas G.T. Jaenson. © World Health Organization 2004
www.who.int/iris/handle/10665/117697 Sponsored by the Vector Biology and Control unit in WHO/EMRO Eastern Mediterranean Health Journal, Vol. 15, No. 3, 2009 761 Case report Congenital tick-borne relapsing fever: report of a case with transplacental transmission in the Islamic Republic of Iran, M. Mahram and M.B. Ghavami. © World Health Organization 2006
http://iris.wpro.who.int/handle/10665.1/7999 REPORT OF THE REGIONAL DIRECTOR
The Work of WHO in the Western Pacific Region 1 July 2011-30 June 2012
http://www.who.int/tdr/stewardship/global_report/en/ Global report for Research Infectious diseases of Poverty 2012 WHO publication. Chapter 1 - Why research infectious diseases of poverty?
http://apps.who.int/iris/bitstream/10665/111008/1/WHO_DCO_WHD_2014.1_ eng.pdf A global brief on vector-borne diseases © World Health Organization 2014

[2] Citation come from CDC. (2013) International Conference on Lyme Borreliosis and other Tick-borne Diseases. 18 Aug 2013

[3] The term Lyme disease typically refers to an infection by Borrelia Burgdorferi, wheras the more term Lyme borreliosis encompasses the different forms of borrelia that cause Lyme disease.

[4] European center for disease control and prevention. Second expert consultation on tick- borne diseases with emphasis on Lyme borreliosis and tick-borne encephalitis. 22-23 November 2011.
Petra Hopf-Siedel, Chronic persistent Lyme disease. August 2012. http://www.borreliose-nachrichten.de/wp- content/uploads/2012/03/Chronic_persistent_Lyme-Disease_or_chronic_Borreliosis.pdf
European commission, Health and consumer directorate-General: Director C- Public health and risk assessment C2- health information on Lyme disease incidences.

[5] Xian-Bo Wu, Ren-Hua Na, Shan-Shan Wei, Jin-Song Zhu and Hong-Juan Peng. Distribution of tick-borne diseases in China, Parasites & Vectors 2013 6:119 DOI: 10.1186/1756-3305-6-119
https://parasitesandvectors.biomedcentral.com/articles/10.1186/1756-3305-6-119

[6] Adrion ER, Aucott J, Lemke KW, Weiner JP. *Health care costs, utilization and patterns of care following Lyme disease.* PLOS ONE. 2015;10(2):e0116767. doi: 10.1371/journal.pone.0116767

[7] DEPARTMENT of HEALTH and HUMAN SERVICES Fiscal Year 2016 Justification of Estimates for Appropriation Committees Page 417 "CDC Performance measure for Long Term Objective: Protect

Americans from Infectious Diseases- Vector-borne. 3.E: Establish state TickNet sites to collect and submit data for Lyme and other tick-borne diseases (Output) 2014 – 2017 Establish state TickNet 16 per year."

[8] Cameron DJ, Johnson LB, Maloney EL. Evidence assessments and guideline recommendations in Lyme disease: The clinical management of known tick bites, erythema migrans rashes and persistent disease. *Expert Review of Anti-infective Therapy*. 2014;12(9):1103-1135. doi:10.1586/14787210.2014.940900

[9] Lyme tests

Cook M, Puri B. Commercial test kits for detection of Lyme borreliosis: A meta-analysis of test accuracy. *International Journal of General Medicine*. 2016; Volume 9:427-440. doi:10.2147/ijgm.s122313

Schwarzwalder A1, Schneider MF, Lydecker A, Aucott JN Sex differences in the clinical and serologic presentation of early Lyme disease: Results from a retrospective review. Gend Med. 2010 Aug;7(4):320-9. doi: 10.1016/j.genm.2010.08.002.

Stricker RB, Johnson L. Let's tackle the testing. *Letter*. 2007;335(7628):1008. doi:10.1136/bmj.39394. 676227.BE. http://dx.doi.org/10.1136/bmj.39394.676227.BE. Accessed February 19, 2017

[10] http://www.ohchr.org/Documents/Publications/Factsheet31.pdf
http://www.ohchr.org/Documents/Issues/ESCR/Health/RightToHealthWHOFS2.pdf

[11] See SDG-HR table: http://www.ohchr.org/Documents/Issues/MDGs/Post2015/SDG_HR_Table.pdf as well as the comment of the Special Rapporteur on the Right to Health about the SDGs: http://www.ifhhro.org/news-a-events/612-the-right-to-health-and-the-sustainable-development-goals

[12] United Nations Office of the Special Advisor on Africa (OSAA) and the NEPAD-OECD Africa Investment Initiative. Africa Fact Sheet Main Economic Indicators, United Nations Office of the Special Adviser on Africa, (2005). https://www.oecd.org/investment/investmentfordevelopment/47452483.pdf

[13] Dworkin MS, Schwan TG, Anderson DE, Borchardt SM. Tick-borne Relapsing fever. *Infectious Disease Clinics of North America*. 2008;22(3):449-468. doi: 10.1016/j.idc.2008.03.006. https://uic.pure.elsevier.com/en/publications/tick-borne- relapsing-fever. Accessed February 19, 2017.

[14] Dupont HT1, La Scola B, Williams R, Raoult D. *A focus of tick-borne relapsing fever in southern Zaire*. Clin Infect Dis. 1997 Jul;25(1):139-44. PMID: 9243047 https://www.ncbi.nlm.nih.gov/pubmed/9243047

[15] Diatta G, Duplantier J-M, Granjon L, et al. *Borrelia infection in small mammals in west Africa and its relationship with tick occurrence inside burrows. Acta Tropica*. 2015;152:131-140. doi:10.1016/j.actatropica.2015.08.016.

[16] EPA, Climate Change Indicators in the United States: Lyme disease. http://www.epa.gov/climatechange/science/indicators/

[17] DellaSala DA, Middelveen M, Liegner KB, Luche-Thayer J. *Lyme disease epidemic increasing globally due to climate change and human activities*. The Encyclopedia of the Anthropocene. in press.

[18] Adrion ER, Aucott J, Lemke KW, Weiner JP. Health Care Costs, Utilization and Patterns of Care following Lyme Disease. 2015. *PLoS ONE* 10(2): e0116767.

[19] http://www.ohchr.org/Documents/Publications/Factsheet31.pdf

[20] https://downloads.globalchange.gov/sap/sap4-6/sap4-6-final-report-all.pdf

[21] https://www.gradeworkinggroup.org/

[22] Magnusson R. *Advancing the right to health: The vital role of law*. Geneva: World Health Organization; 2017. http://apps.who.int/iris/bitstream/10665/252815/1/9789241511384- eng.pdf. Accessed February 15, 2017.

[23] Standards Committee, Institute of Medicine, Board on Health Care Services. *Clinical practice guidelines we can trust*. Graham R, Mancher M, Miller Wolman D, Greenfield S, Steinberg E, eds. Washington, DC: National Academies Press; June 16, 2011

[24] From a March 2017 interview by the *On Lyme Foundation* with BVIZK chairman Vera Hooglugt.

[25] The principal author of the report has permission to publicize Teike's situation and has determined to limit the sharing of his personal information in this report. The laboratory that provided the Lyme borrelia and bartonella testing service is solidly legitimate; for example, this lab was one of the selected collaborators for the European Union's scientific research program's Hilysens project. Requests for more details of this shameful case can be sent to the principal author.

References include: (1) Buiting H, van Delden J, Onwuteaka-Philpsen B, et al. (2009). "Reporting of euthanasia and physician-assisted suicide in the Netherlands: descriptive study". BMC Med Ethics. 10: 18. doi:10.1186/1472-6939-10-18. PMC 2781018Freely accessible. PMID 19860873.

(2) Rietjens JA, van der Maas PJ, Onwuteaka-Philipsen BD, van Delden JJ, van der Heide A (September 2009). "Two Decades of Research on Euthanasia from the Netherlands. What Have We Learnt and What Questions Remain?". J Bioeth Inq. 6 (3): 271-283. doi:10.1007/s11673-009-9172-3. PMC 2733179Freely accessible. PMID 19718271.

[26] Burgdorfer W. Discovery of the Lyme disease spirochete and its relation to tick vectors. *The Yale journal of biology and medicine*. 1984;57(4):515-20. https://www.ncbi.nlm.nih.gov/pubmed/6516454. Accessed February 19, 2017

[27] Steere A, Malawista S, Snydman D, et al. Lyme arthritis: An epidemic of oligoarticular arthritis in children and adults in three Connecticut communities. *Arthritis and rheumatism*. 1977;20(1):7-17. https://www.ncbi.nlm.nih.gov/pubmed/836338. Accessed February 19, 2017

[28] Mannelli A, Bertolotti L, Gern L, Gray J. Ecology of Borrelia burgdorferi sensu lato in Europe: Transmission dynamics in multi-host systems, influence of molecular processes and effects of climate change. FEMS Microbiology Reviews. 2012;36(4):837-861. doi:10.1111/j.1574-6976.2011.00312.x.

[29] McManus M, Cincotta A. Effects of Borrelia on host immune system: Possible consequences for diagnostics. Advances in Integrative Medicine. 2015;2(2):81-89. doi:10.1016/j.aimed.2014.11.002

[30] Rudenko N, Golovchenko M, Grubhoffer L, Oliver JH. Updates on Borrelia burgdorferi sensu lato complex with respect to public health. *Ticks and Tick-borne Diseases*. 2011;2(3):123-128. doi:10.1016/j.ttbdis.2011.04.002.

[31] Cutler SJ1, Rudenko N2, Golovchenko M2, Cramaro WJ3, Kirpach J3, Savic S4, Christova I5, Amaro A6. Diagnosing Borreliosis. Vector Borne Zoonotic Dis. 2017 Jan;17(1):2-11. doi: 10.1089/vbz.2016.1962.

Rudenko N, Golovchenko M, Grubhoffer L, Oliver JH. Updates on Borrelia burgdorferi sensu lato complex with respect to public health. *Ticks and Tick-borne Diseases*. 2011;2(3):123-128. doi: 10.1016/j.ttbdis.2011.04.002

Qiu WG, Martin CL. Evolutionary genomics of borrelia burgdorferi sensu lato: findings, hypotheses, and the rise of hybrids. Infect Genet Evol. 2014;27C:576-93

Qiu W-G, Schutzer SE, Bruno JF, et al. Genetic exchange and plasmid transfers in Borrelia burgdorferi sensu stricto revealed by three-way genome comparisons and multilocus sequence typing. Proceedings of the National Academy of Sciences of the United States of America. 2004;101(39):14150-14155. doi:10.1073/pnas.0402745101. http://www.pnas.org/content/101/39/14150.long. Accessed February 18, 2017.

[32] Berndtson K. Review of evidence for immune evasion and persistent infection in Lyme | IJGM. *International Journal of General Medicine*. 2013; Volume 6:291-306. doi: 10.2147/IJGM.S44114. http://dx.doi.org/10.2147/IJGM.S44114. Accessed February 19, 2017

[33] Kumar Singh S, Josef Girschick H. Molecualar survival strategies of the Lyme disease spirochete Borrelia burgdorferi. The Lancet Infectious Diseases. 2004;4(9):575-583. doi:10.1016/s1473-3099(04)01132-6

Hovius JWR, van Dam AP, Fikrig E. Tick-host-pathogen interactions in Lyme borreliosis. Trends in Parasitology. 2007;23(9):434-438. doi:10.1016/j.pt.2007.07.001.

Fikrig E, Narasimhan S. Borrelia burgdorferi-Traveling incognito? Microbes and Infection. 2006;8(5):1390-1399. doi: 10.1016/j.micinf.2005.12.022.

Kraiczy P. Hide and seek: How Lyme disease Spirochetes overcome complement attack. Frontiers in Immunology. 2016;7. doi:10.3389/fimmu.2016.00385.

Wu Q, Guan G, Liu Z, Li Y, Luo J, Yin H. RNA-Seq-based analysis of changes in Borrelia burgdorferi gene expression linked to pathogenicity. Parasites & Vectors. 2015;8(1):155. doi:10.1186/s13071-014-0623-2.

Feng J, Shi W, Zhang S, Zhang Y. Persister mechanisms in Borrelia burgdorferi: Implications for improved intervention. Emerging Microbes & Infections. 2015;4(8):e51. doi:10.1038/emi.2015.51.

[34] Alban PS, Nelson DR, Johnson PW. Serum-starvation-induced changes in protein synthesis and morphology of Borrelia burgdorferi. *Microbiology*. 2000;146(1):119-127. doi:10.1099/00221287-146-1-119.

BRORSON Ø, BRORSON S-H. A rapid method for generating cystic forms ofBorrelia burgdorferi, and their reversal to mobile spirochetes. *APMIS*. 1998;106(7-12):1131-1141. doi:10.1111/j.1699-0463.1998.tb00269.x.

Gruntar I, Malovrh T, Murgia R, Cinco M. Conversion of Borrelia garinii cystic forms to motile spirochetes in vivoNote. *APMIS*. 2001;109(5):383-388. doi:10.1034/j.1600-0463.2001.090507.x.

Hodzic E, Imai D, Feng S, Barthold SW. Resurgence of persisting Non-Cultivable Borrelia burgdorferi following antibiotic treatment in mice. *PLoS ONE*. 2014;9(1):e86907. doi: 10.1371/journal.pone.0086907.

Sharma B, Brown AV, Matluck NE, Hu LT, Lewis K. Borrelia burgdorferi, the causative agent of Lyme disease, forms drug-tolerant Persister cells. *Antimicrobial Agents and Chemotherapy*. 2015;59(8):4616-4624. doi:10.1128/aac.00864-15.

[35] Pausa M, Pellis V, Cinco M, et al. Serum-resistant strains of Borrelia burgdorferi evade complement-mediated killing by expressing a CD59-Like complement inhibitory molecule. *The Journal of Immunology*. 2003;170(6):3214-3222. doi:10.4049/jimmunol.170.6.3214

[36] Bockenstedt LK, Gonzalez DG, Haberman AM, Belperron AA. Spirochete antigens persist near cartilage after murine Lyme borreliosis therapy. *The Journal of Clinical Investigation*. 2012;122(7):2652-2660. doi:10.1172/JCI58813. http://dx.doi.org/10.1172/JCI58813. Accessed February 19, 2017.

Chary-Valckenaere I. Ultrastructural demonstration of intracellular localization of Borrelia burgdorferi in Lyme arthritis. *Rheumatology*. 1998; 37(4):468-470. doi: 10.1093/rheumatology/37.4.468.

Coyle PK, Schutzer SE, Deng Z, et al. Detection of Borrelia burgdorferi-specific antigen in antibody-negative cerebrospinal fluid in neurologic Lyme disease. *Neurology*. 1995; 45(11):2010-2015. doi: 10.1212/wnl.45.11.2010.

Coyle PK, Deng Z, Schutzer SE, et al. Detection of Borrelia burgdorferi antigens in cerebrospinal fluid. *Neurology*. 1993;43(6):1093-1093. doi:10.1212/wnl.43.6.1093.

Embers ME, Barthold SW, Borda JT, et al. Persistence of Borrelia burgdorferi in Rhesus Macaques following antibiotic treatment of disseminated infection. *PLoS ONE*. 2012;7(1):e29914. doi: 10.1371/journal.pone.0029914.

Feng J, Weitner M, Shi W, Zhang S, Zhang Y. Eradication of Biofilm-Like Microcolony structures of Borrelia burgdorferi by Daunomycin and Daptomycin but not Mitomycin C in combination with Doxycycline and Cefuroxime. *Frontiers in Microbiology*. 2016;7. doi:10.3389/fmicb.2016.00062.

Feng J, Zhang S, Shi W, Zhang Y. Ceftriaxone pulse Dosing fails to eradicate Biofilm-Like Microcolony B. Burgdorferi Persisters which are sterilized by Daptomycin/ Doxycycline/Cefuroxime without pulse Dosing. *Frontiers in Microbiology*. 2016;7. doi:10.3389/fmicb.2016.01744.

Häupl T, Hahn G, Rittig M, et al. Persistence of Borrelia burgdorferi in ligamentous tissue from a patient with chronic Lyme borreliosis. *Arthritis and rheumatism*. 1993;36(11):1621-6. https://www.ncbi.nlm.nih.gov/pubmed/8240439. Accessed February 19, 2017.

Hodzic E, Feng S, Holden K, Freet KJ, Barthold SW. Persistence of Borrelia burgdorferi following antibiotic treatment in mice. *Antimicrobial Agents and Chemotherapy*.

2008;52(5):1728-1736. doi:10.1128/aac.01050-07.

Hodzic E, Imai D, Feng S, Barthold SW. Resurgence of persisting Non-Cultivable Borrelia burgdorferi following antibiotic treatment in mice. *PLoS ONE*. 2014;9(1):e86907. doi: 10.1371/journal.pone.0086907.

Marques A, Telford SR, Turk S, et al. Xenodiagnosis to detect Borrelia burgdorferi infection: A First-in-Human study. *Clinical Infectious Diseases*. 2014;58(7):937-945. doi:10.1093/cid/cit939.

Miklossy J, Khalili K, Gern L, et al. Borrelia burgdorferi persists in the brain in chronic lyme neuroborreliosis and may be associated with Alzheimer disease. *Journal of Alzheimer's disease: JAD*. 2005;6(6):639-49. https://www.ncbi.nlm.nih.gov/pubmed/15665404. Accessed February 19, 2017.

Miklossy J, Kasas S, Zurn AD, McCall S, Yu S, McGeer PL. Persisting atypical and cystic forms of Borrelia burgdorferi and local inflammation in Lyme neuroborreliosis. *Journal of Neuroinflammation*. 2008;5(1):40. doi:10.1186/1742-2094-5-40.

Muehlenbachs A, Bollweg BC, Schulz TJ, et al. Cardiac Tropism of Borrelia burgdorferi. *The American Journal of Pathology*. 2016;186(5):1195-1205. doi: 10.1016/j.ajpath.2015.12.027.

Oksi J, Kalimo H, Marttila R, et al. Inflammatory brain changes in Lyme borreliosis. A report on three patients and review of literature. *Brain: a journal of neurology*. 1996; 119:2143-54. https://www.ncbi.nlm.nih.gov/pubmed/9010017. Accessed February 19, 2017.

Preac-Mursic V, Weber K, Pfister H, et al. Survival of Borrelia burgdorferi in antibiotically treated patients with Lyme borreliosis. *Infection*. 1989;17(6):355-9. https://www.ncbi.nlm.nih.gov/pubmed/2613324. Accessed February 19, 2017.

Rudenko N, Golovchenko M, Mokracek A, et al. Detection of Borrelia bissettii in cardiac valve tissue of a patient with Endocarditis and Aortic valve Stenosis in the Czech Republic. *Journal of Clinical Microbiology*. 2008;46(10):3540-3543. doi:10.1128/jcm.01032-08.

Rudenko N, Golovchenko M, Vancova M, Clark K, Grubhoffer L, Oliver JH. Isolation of live Borrelia burgdorferi sensu lato spirochaetes from patients with undefined disorders and symptoms not typical for Lyme borreliosis. *Clinical Microbiology and Infection*. 2016;22(3): 267.e9-267.e15. doi: 10.1016/j.cmi.2015.11.009.

Sapi E, Balasubramanian K, Poruri A, et al. Evidence of in vivo existence of Borrelia biofilm in borrelial lymphocytomas. *European Journal of Microbiology and Immunology*. 2016;6(1):9-24. doi:10.1556/1886.2015.00049.

Sharma B, Brown AV, Matluck NE, Hu LT, Lewis K. Borrelia burgdorferi, the causative agent of Lyme disease, forms drug-tolerant Persister cells. *Antimicrobial Agents and Chemotherapy*. 2015;59(8):4616-4624. doi:10.1128/aac.00864-15.

Singh SK, Girschick HJ. Molecualar survival strategies of the Lyme disease spirochete Borrelia burgdorferi. *The Lancet Infectious Diseases*. 2004;4(9):575-583. doi:10.1016/s1473- 3099(04)01132-6.

Straubinger R, Summers B, Chang Y, Appel M. Persistence of Borrelia burgdorferi in experimentally infected dogs after antibiotic treatment. *Journal of clinical microbiology*. 1997;35(1):111-6. https://www.ncbi.nlm.nih.gov/pubmed/8968890. Accessed February 19, 2017.

[37] Rudenko N, Golovchenko M, Grubhoffer L, Oliver JH. Updates on Borrelia burgdorferi sensu lato complex with respect to public health. *Ticks and Tick-borne Diseases*. 2011;2(3):123- 128. doi:10.1016/j.ttbdis.2011.04.002

[38] Batinac T, Petranovic D, Zamolo G, Ruzic A. Lyme borreliosis and multiple sclerosis are associated with primary effusion lymphoma. *Medical Hypotheses*. 2007;69(1):117-119. doi:10.1016/j.mehy.2006.11.015

[39] Zanchi AC, Gingold AR, Theise ND, Min AD. Necrotizing Granulomatous hepatitis as an unusual manifestation of Lyme disease. *Digestive Diseases and Sciences*. 2007;52(10):2629- 2632. doi:10.1007/s10620-006-9405-9.

40 Garbe C, Stein H, Dienemann D, Orfanos CE. Borrelia burgdorferi—associated cutaneous B cell lymphoma: Clinical and immunohistologic characterization of four cases. *Journal of the American Academy of Dermatology*. 1991;24(4):584-590. doi:10.1016/0190-9622(91)70088-j.

41 Psychiatric complications

Fallon BA, Kochevar JM, Gaito A, Nields JA. The underdiagnosis of neuropsychiatric lyme disease in children and adults. *Psychiatric Clinics of North America*. 1998;21(3):693-703. doi:10.1016/s0193-953x(05)70032-0.

Fallon BA, Schwartzberg M, Bransfield R, et al. Late-stage neuropsychiatric Lyme Borreliosis. *Psychosomatics*. 1995;36(3):295-300. doi:10.1016/s0033-3182(95)71669-3.

Fallon BA, Das S, Plutchok JJ, Tager F, Liegner K, Van Heertum R. Functional brain imaging and Neuropsychological testing in Lyme disease. *Clinical Infectious Diseases*. 1997;25(s1): S57-S63. doi:10.1086/516175.

Fallon BA. Regional cerebral blood flow and cognitive deficits in chronic Lyme disease. *Journal of Neuropsychiatry*. 2003;15(3):326-332. doi:10.1176/appi.neuropsych.15.3.326.

42 Walther EU, Seelos K, Bise K, Mayer M, Straube A. Lyme Neuroborreliosis mimicking primary CNS lymphoma. *European Neurology*. 2004;51(1):43-45. doi:10.1159/000075086

43 Immune dysregulation

Aberer E1, Koszik F, Silberer M. Why is chronic Lyme borreliosis chronic? Clin Infect Dis. 1997 Jul;25 Suppl 1: S64-70. http://www.ncbi.nlm.nih.gov/pubmed/9233667

Cabral ES1, Gelderblom H, Hornung RL, Munson PJ, Martin R, Marques AR. Borrelia burgdorferi lipoprotein-mediated TLR2 stimulation causes the down-regulation of TLR5 in human monocytes. J Infect Dis. 2006 Mar 15;193(6):849-59. Epub 2006 Feb 8. http://www.ncbi.nlm.nih.gov/pubmed/16479520

Cassiani-Ingoni R1, Cabral ES, Lünemann JD, Garza Z, Magnus T, Gelderblom H, Munson PJ, Marques A, Martin R. Borrelia burgdorferi Induces TLR1 and TLR2 in human microglia and peripheral blood monocytes but differentially regulates HLA-class II expression. J Neuropathol Exp Neurol. 2006 Jun;65(6):540-8. http://www.ncbi.nlm.nih.gov/pubmed/16988256

Chiao JW, Pavia C, Riley M, Altmann-Lasekan W, Abolhassani M, Liegner K, Mittelman A. Antigens of Lyme disease of spirochaete Borrelia burgdorferi inhibits antigen or mitogen- induced lymphocyte proliferation. FEMS Immunol Med Microbiol. 1994 Feb;8(2):151-5. http://www.ncbi.nlm.nih.gov/pubmed/8173554

Chiao JW1, Villalon P, Schwartz I, Wormser GP. Modulation of lymphocyte proliferative responses by a canine Lyme disease vaccine of recombinant outer surface protein A (OspA). FEMS Immunol Med Microbiol. 2000 Jul;28(3):193-6. http://www.ncbi.nlm.nih.gov/pubmed/10865170

Diterich I1, Rauter C, Kirschning CJ, Hartung T. Borrelia burgdorferi-induced tolerance as a model of persistence via immunosuppression. Infect Immun. 2003 Jul;71(7):3979-87. http://www.ncbi.nlm.nih.gov/pubmed/12819085

Durovska J1, Bazovska S, Ondrisova M, Pancak J. Our experience with examination of antibodies against antigens of Borrelia burgdorferi in patients with suspected lyme disease. Bratisl Lek Listy. 2010;111(3):153-5. http://www.ncbi.nlm.nih.gov/pubmed/20437826

Elsner RA1, Hastey CJ1, Baumgarth N2CD4+ T cells promote antibody production but not sustained affinity maturation during Borrelia burgdorferi infection. Infect Immun. 2015 Jan;83(1):48-56. doi: 10.1128/IAI.02471-14. http://www.ncbi.nlm.nih.gov/pubmed/25312948

Elsner RA, Hastey CJ, Olsen KJ, Baumgarth N (2015) Suppression of Long-Lived Humoral Immunity Following Borrelia burgdorferi Infection. PLoS Pathog 11(7) : e1004976. doi:10.1371/journal.ppat.1004976 http://journals.plos.org/plospathogens/article?id=10.1371/journal.ppat.1004976

Ganapamo F1, Dennis VA, Philipp MT. Early induction of gamma interferon and interleukin-10 production in draining lymph nodes from mice infected with Borrelia burgdorferi. Infect Immun. 2000 Dec;68(12):7162-5. http://www.ncbi.nlm.nih.gov/pubmed/11083848

Gautam A1, Dixit S, Philipp MT, Singh SR, Morici LA, Kaushal D, Dennis VA. Interleukin-10 alters effector functions of multiple genes induced by Borrelia burgdorferi in macrophages to regulate Lyme disease inflammation. Infect Immun. 2011 Dec;79(12):4876-92. doi: 10.1128/IAI.05451-11. Epub 2011 Sep 26. http://www.ncbi.nlm.nih.gov/pubmed/21947773

Gautam A1, Dixit S, Embers M, Gautam R, Philipp MT, Singh SR, Morici L, Dennis Different patterns of expression and of IL-10 modulation of inflammatory mediators from macrophages of Lyme disease-resistant and -susceptible mice. PLoS One. 2012;7(9):e43860. Epub 2012 Sep 14. http://www.ncbi.nlm.nih.gov/pubmed/23024745

Guillermo H. Giambartolomei, Vida A. Dennis, * and Mario T. Philipp. Borrelia burgdorferi Stimulates the Production of Interleukin-10 in Peripheral Blood Mononuclear Cells from Uninfected Humans and Rhesus Monkeys. Infect Immun. 1998 Jun; 66(6): 2691-2697. http://www.ncbi.nlm.nih.gov/pmc/articles/PMC108257

Hulínská D1, Roubalová K, Schramlová J. Interaction of Borrelia burgdorferi sensu lato with Epstein-Barr virus in lymphoblastoid cells. Folia Biol (Praha). 2003;49(1):40-8. http://www.ncbi.nlm.nih.gov/pubmed/12630667

Jarefors S1, Janefjord CK, Forsberg P, Jenmalm MC, Ekerfelt C. Decreased up-regulation of the interleukin-12Rbeta2-chain and interferon-gamma secretion and increased number of forkhead box P3-expressing cells in patients with a history of chronic Lyme borreliosis compared with asymptomatic Borrelia-exposed individuals. Clin Exp Immunol. 2007 Jan;147(1):18-27. http://www.ncbi.nlm.nih.gov/pubmed/17177959

John J. Lazarus, Maria A. Kay, Akisha L. McCarter, and R. Mark Wooten. Viable Borrelia burgdorferi Enhances Interleukin-10 Production and Suppresses Activation of Murine Macrophages. Infect Immun. 2008 Mar; 76(3): 1153–1162. http://www.ncbi.nlm.nih.gov/pmc/articles/PMC2258815

Tunev SS, Hastey CJ, Hodzic E, Feng S, Barthold SW, Baumgarth N (2011) Lymphoadenopathy during Lyme Borreliosis Is Caused by Spirochete Migration-Induced Specific B Cell Activation. PLoS Pathog 7(5) : e1002066. doi: 10.1371/journal.ppat.1002066. http://journals.plos.org/plospathogens/article?id=10.1371/journal.ppat.1002066

Yutein Chung, Nan Zhang, and R. Mark Wooden. Borrelia burgdorferi Elicited-IL-10 Suppresses the Production of Inflammatory Mediators, Phagocytosis, and Expression of Co- Stimulatory Receptors by Murine Macrophages and/or Dendritic Cells. PLoS One. 2014; 9(1): 10.1371/annotation/680090aa-3e1b-4135-94d6-8082c09180d4. http://www.ncbi.nlm.nih.gov/pmc/articles/PMC3868605

[44] Zaidi, Syed Ali, and Carol Singer. 2002. "Gastrointestinal and Hepatic Manifestations of Tickborne Diseases in the United States." Clinical Infectious Diseases 34 (9): 1206–12. http://dx.doi.org/10.1086/339871

[45] Mark S. Dworkin, MD, MPH TM,a,* Tom G. Schwan, PhD,b Donald E. Anderson, Jr, PhD,c and Stephanie M. Borchardt, PhD, MPHd *Tick-Borne Relapsing Fever* Infect Dis Clin North Am. Author manuscript; available in PMC 2013 Jul 29. Published in final edited form as: Infect Dis Clin North Am. 2008 Sep; 22(3): 449–viii. doi: 10.1016/j.idc.2008.03.006 PMCID: PMC3725823 NIHMSID: NIHMS492680 www.ncbi.nlm.nih.gov/pmc/articles/PMC3725823/

[46] Coinfections

Dr.'s Eskow/Mordechai et.al.; Concurrent infection of the Central Nervous System by Borrelia burgorferi and Bartonella henselae. Archives of Neurology Sept 2001

Hofmeister et.al.; A Novel Bartonella species in Peromyscus leucopus in conjunction with B. burgdorferi and Babesia microti. J. Infect Disease 1998

Lebech et al. Serologic evidence of granulocytic ehrlichiosis and piroplasma WA 1 in European patients with Lyme neuroborreliosis. Seventh Intl Congress on Lyme Borreliosis 1996:390

Minar et al. Natural foci of tick-borne encephalitis in central Europe and the relationship of the incidence of Ixodes ricinus to original ecosystems. Cent Eur J Public Health 1995;3:337

© Copyright 2017 Global Network on Institutional Discrimination and the Ad Hoc Committee for Health Equity in ICD11 Borreliosis Codes. All Rights reserved

Rafal Tokarz, Komal Jain, Ashlee Bennett, Thomas Briese, and W. Ian Lipkin. Assessment of Polymicrobial Infections in Ticks in New York State *Vector Borne Zoonotic* Dis. 2010 Apr; 10(3): 217-221. doi: 10.1089/vbz.2009.0036 PMCID: PMC2883481

Schoub et.al.; High Percentage of Ixodes ricinus ticks are co-infected with Borrelia, Ehrlichia, and Bartonella (Netherlands). J. Clin Microbiology 1999; (37:2215-2215)

[47] SH Lee, et al. Detection of Borreliae in Archived Sera from Patients with Clinically Suspect Lyme Disease. Int. J. Mol. Sci. 2014, 15(3), 4284-4298

[48] Grankvist A, Sandelin L, Andersson J, et al. Infections with Candidatus Neoehrlichia mikurensis and Cytokine Responses in 2 Persons Bitten by Ticks, Sweden. Emerging Infectious Diseases. 2015;21(8):1462-1465. doi:10.3201/eid2108.150060. *and references therein*

[49] https://jneuroinflammation.biomedcentral.com/articles/10.1186/1742-2094-8-90
Miklossy J. Alzheimer's disease - a neurospirochetosis. Analysis of the evidence following Koch's and Hill's criteria. Neuroinflammation. 2011 Aug 4;8:90. doi: 10.1186/1742-2094-8-90.

https://www.ncbi.nlm.nih.gov/pubmed/21816039
Miklossy J. Biology and neuropathology of dementia in syphilis and Lyme disease. In: Handbook of Clinical Neurology, Dementias, Vol 89 (3rd series), Eds: C Duyckaerts, I Litvan, Elsevier, (Edinburgh, London, New York, Oxford, Philadelphia, St-Louis, Toronto, Sydney) Series Eds : MJ Aminoff, F Boller, DS Schwab), 2008, Volume 89, Chapter 72, pp. 825-844.

[50] Forrester, Joseph D, and Paul Mead. 2014. "Third-Degree Heart Block Associated With Lyme Carditis: Review of Published Cases." *Clinical Infectious Diseases* 59 (7): 996–1000.
http://dx.doi.org/10.1093/cid/ciu411

[51] arthritis

Albert S, Schulze J, Riegel H, Brade V. Lyme arthritis in a 12-year-old patient after a latency period of 5 years. Infection 1999; 27(4-5): 286-288.

Battafarano DF, Combs JA, Enzenauer RJ, Fitzpatrick JE. Chronic septic arthritis caused by Borrelia burgdorferi. Clin Orthop 1993; 297: 238-241.

Chary-Valckenaere I, Jaulhac B, Champigneulle J, Piement Y, Mainard D, and Pourel J. Ultrastructural demonstration of intracellular localization of Borrelia burgdorferi in Lyme arthritis. Br J Rheumatol 1998; 37: 468-470.

Dejmková H, D Hulinska, D Tegzová, K Pavelka, J Gatterová, and P Vavřik. Seronegative Lyme arthritis caused by Borrelia garinii. Clin Rheumatol 2002; 21:330-334.

Franz JK, O Fritze, M Rittig et al. Insights from a novel three-dimensional in vitro model of Lyme arthritis: standardized analysis of cellular and molecular interactions between Borrelia burgdorferi and synovial explants and fibroblasts. Arthritis Rheum 2001; 44: 151-162.

Holl-Weiden A, Suerbaum S, and Girschick HJ. Seronegative Lyme arthritis. Rheumatology International 2007; 11: 1091-1093.

Marlovits S, Khanah G, Striessniq G, Vécsei V, and Stanek G. Emergence of Lyme arthritis after autologous chondrocyte transplantation. Arthritis Rheum. 2004; 50: 259-264.

Nocton JJ, Dressler F, Rutledge BJ, Rys PN, Persing DH, and Steere AC. Detection of Borrelia burgdorferi DNA by polymerase chain reaction in synovial fluid from patients with Lyme arthritis. N Eng J Med 1994; 330: 229-234.

Schoen RT, Aversa JM, Rahn DW, and Steere AC. Treatment of refractory chronic Lyme arthritis with arthroscopic synvectomy. Arthritis Rheum 1991; 34(8): 1056-1060.

Yang L, Weis JH, Eichwald E, Kolbert CP, Persing DH, and Weis JJ. Heritable susceptibility to severe Borrelia burgdorferi-induced arthritis is dominant and is associated with persistence of large numbers of spirochetes in tissues. Infect Immun 1994; 62: 492-500.

[52] Loss of hearing

Bertholon P. Sensorineural hearing loss: a complex feature in Lyme disease. Otol Neurotol. 2013 Oct;34(8):1543. doi: 10.1097/MAO.0b013e3182a007d4. No abstract available. PMID: 24005168

Maniu A, Damian L. Rapid progressive bilateral hearing loss due to granulomatous otitis media in Lyme disease. Am J Otolaryngol. 2013 May-Jun;34(3):245-7. doi: 10.1016/j.amjoto.2012.11.009. PMID: 23313123

[53] Sathiamoorthi, S. and W.M. Smith, The eye and tick-borne disease in the United States. Curr Opin Ophthalmol, 2016. 27(6): p. 530-537.

[54] dementia

Miklossy J. Alzheimer's disease — a spirochetosis? NeuroReport 1993; 4: 841-848.

Miklossy J, Kasas S, Janzer RC, Ardizzoni F, and Loos H. Further morphological evidence of a spirochetal etiology of Alzheimer's disease. NeuroReport 1994; 5: 1201-1204.

Miklossy J, Gern L, Darekar P, Janzer RC, Loos H. Senile plaques, neurofibrillary tangles and neuropil threads contain DNA? J Spirochetal and Tick-borne Dis 1995; 2: 1-5.

Miklossy JM, Khalili K, Gern L, Ericson RL, Darekar P, Bolle L, Hurlimann J, and Paster BJ. Borrelia burgdorferi persists in the brain in chronic Lyme neuroborreliosis and may be associated with Alzheimer's disease. J Alzheimers Dis 2004; 6; 639-649.

Miklossy J, Rosemberg S, and McGeer PL; Beta amyloid deposition in the atrophic form of general paresis. In Alzheimer's Disease: New advances. Medimond. Proceedings of the 10th International Congress on Alzheimer's Disease. Edited by: Iqbal K, Winblad B, and Avila J; 2006: 429-433.

Miklossy J, Kris A, Radenovic A, Miller L, Forro L, Martins R, Reiss K, Darbinian N, Darekara P, Mihaly L, and Khalili K. Beta amyloid deposition and Alzheimer's type changes induced by Borrelia spirochetes. Neurobiol Aging 2006; 27: 228-236.

Miklossy J. Chronic inflammation and amyloidogenesis in Alzheimer's disease — role of spirochetes. J Alzheimers Dis 2008; 13: 381-391.

Miklossy, J. 2008. Biology and neuropathology of dementia in syphilis and Lyme disease. In Handbook of Clinical Neurology, Vol. 89. C. Duyckaerts, I. Litvan (eds.). Elsevier, Amsterdam, Netherlands. p. 825-844.

MacDonald AB. In situ DNA hybridization study of granulovacuolar degeneration in human Alzheimer autopsy neurons for flagellin b transcriptomes of Borrelia burgdorferi. Alzheimer's Dis Dementia 2006; 2 (Suppl. 1): S207.

MacDonald AB. Cystic borrelia in Alzheimer's disease and in non-dementia neuroborreliosis. Alzheimer's Dementia 2006; 2 (Suppl. 1): S433.

Waniek C, Prohovnik I, Kaufman MA, and Dwork AJ. Rapid progressive frontal-type dementia associated with Lyme disease. J Neuropsychiatry Clin Neurosci 1995; 7: 345-347. (B. burgdorferi detected at autopsy).

[55] Strokes

Back T1, Grünig S, Winter Y, Bodechtel U, Guthke K, Khati D, von Kummer R. Neuroborreliosis-associated cerebral vasculitis: long-term outcome and health-related quality of life. J Neurol. 2013 Jun;260(6):1569-75. doi: 10.1007/s00415-013-6831-4. Epub 2013 Jan 18.
https://www.ncbi.nlm.nih.gov/pubmed/23329377

Zajkowska J1, Garkowski A, Moniuszko A, Czupryna P, Ptaszyńska-Sarosiek I, Tarasów E, Ustymowicz A, Łebkowski W, Pancewicz S. Vasculitis and stroke due to Lyme neuroborreliosis - a review. Infect Dis (Lond). 2015 Jan;47(1):1-6. doi: 10.3109/00365548.2014.961544. Epub 2014 Oct 24.
https://www.ncbi.nlm.nih.gov/pubmed/25342573

[56] Zaidi, Syed Ali, and Carol Singer. 2002. "Gastrointestinal and Hepatic Manifestations of Tickborne Diseases in the United States." Clinical Infectious Diseases 34 (9): 1206-12.
http://dx.doi.org/10.1086/339871

57   Finsterer J, Grisold W. Disorders of the lower cranial nerves. Journal of Neurosciences in Rural Practice. 2015;6(3):377-391. doi:10.4103/0976-3147.158768.

58   http://www.cmt.com/news/1768479/kris-kristoffersons-wife-talks-about-misdiagnosis-of-lyme-disease/
http://www.nextavenue.org/kris-kristoffersons-dementia-now-believed-caused-lyme-disease/
http://www.cbsnews.com/news/kris-kristofferson-misdiagnosed-alzheimers-has-lyme-disease/

59   http://www.nytimes.com/health/guides/disease/lyme-disease/print.html

60   Barskova, V G, E S Fedorov, and L P Ananieva. 1999. "The Course of Lyme Disease in Different Age Groups." Wiener Klinische Wochenschrift 111 (22-23 A): 978–80.
http://www.embase.com/search/results?subaction=viewrecord&from=export&id=L30026419%5Cnhttp://rc5hy6jd4f.search.serialssolutions.com?sid=EMBASE&issn=00435325&id=doi:&atitle=The+course+of+Lyme+disease+in+different+age+groups&stitle=Wien.+Klin.+Wochenschr.&titl

61   https://www.cdc.gov/std/syphilis/stdfact-syphilis.htm;
https://www.ncbi.nlm.nih.gov/pubmed/3190104

62   Miklossy J. Biology and neuropathology of dementia in syphilis and Lyme disease. In: Handbook of Clinical Neurology, Dementias, Vol 89 (3rd series), Eds: C Duyckaerts, I Litvan, Elsevier, (Edinburgh, London, New York, Oxford, Philadelphia, St-Louis, Toronto, Sydney) Series Eds: MJ Aminoff, F Boller, DS Schwab), 2008, Volume 89, Chapter 72, pp. 825-844.

63   Congenital Lyme disease, Borrelia *burgdorferi* can potentially infect the fetus and cause adverse fetal outcomes.

Bale JF, Murph JR. Congenital infections and the nervous system. Pediatric Clinics of North America. 1992;39(4):669–690. doi:10.1016/s0031-3955(16)38370-5.

Brzostek T. [Human granulocytic ehrlichiosis co-incident with Lyme borreliosis in pregnant woman--a case study] [in Polish] Przegl Epidemiol. 2004;58(2):289–94.

Gardner T. Lyme disease. In: Remington JS, Klein JO, eds. Infectious Diseases of the Fetus and Newborn. 5th ed. Philadelphia: Saunders; 1995:447–528chap 11.

Gardner T. Lyme disease. In: Remington JS, Klein JO. Infectious diseases of the fetus and newborn infant. 4th ed. Philadelphia: W B Saunders Co; December 13, 1994.

Goldenberg RL, Thompson C. The infectious origins of stillbirth. American Journal of Obstetrics and Gynecology. 2003;189(3):861–873. doi:10.1067/s0002-9378(03)00470-8.

Gustafson JM, Burgess EC, Wachal MD, Steinberg H. Intrauterine transmission of Borrelia burgdorferi in dogs. American Journal of Veterinary Research. 1993;54(6):882–890.

MacDonald AB, Benach JL, Burgdorfer W. Stillbirth following maternal Lyme disease. N Y State J Med. 1987; 11:615–616.

MacDonald AB. Gestational Lyme borreliosis. Implications for the fetus. Rheum Dis Clin North Am. 1989;15(4):657–677.

Macdonald AB. Human fetal borreliosis, toxemia of pregnancy, and fetal death. Zentralblatt für Bakteriologie, Mikrobiologie und Hygiene. Series A: Medical Microbiology, Infectious Diseases, Virology, Parasitology. 1986;263(1-2):189–200. doi:10.1016/s0176- 6724(86)80122-5.

Maraspin V, Cimperman J, Lotric-Furlan S, Pleterski-Rigler D, Strle F. Erythema migrans in pregnancy. Wiener klinische Wochenschrift. 2000; 111:933–40.

Markowitz LE, Steere AC, Benach JL, Slade JD, Broome CV. Lyme disease during pregnancy. JAMA: The Journal of the American Medical Association. 1986;255(24):3394. doi:10.1001/jama.1986.03370240064038.

Schlesinger PA, Duray PH, Burke BA, Steere AC, Stillman MT. Maternal-fetal transmission of the Lyme disease Spirochete, Borrelia burgdorferi. Annals of Internal Medicine. 1985;103(1):67. doi:10.7326/0003-4819-103-1-67.

Silver RM, Yang L, Daynes RA, Branch WD, Salafia CM, Weis JJ. Fetal outcome in Murine Lyme disease. Infection and Immunity. 1995;63(1):66-72.

Strobino BA, Williams CL, Abid S, Ghalson R, Spierling P. Lyme disease and pregnancy outcome: A prospective of two thousand prenatal patients. American Journal of Obstetrics and Gynecology. 1993;169(2):367-374. doi:10.1016/0002-9378(93)90088-z.

Weber K, Bratzke H-J, Neubert U, Wilske B, Duray PH. Borrelia burgdorferi in a newborn despite oral penicillin for Lyme borreliosis during pregnancy. The Pediatric Infectious Disease Journal. 1988;7(4):286-288. doi:10.1097/00006454-198804000-00010.

[64] http://www.who.int/hhr/Economic_social_cultural.pdf

[65] http://www.who.int/medicines/areas/rational_use/en/

[66] One example of stakeholder engagement follows; there are many:

"More than 450 individuals and institutions from around the world attended the ICD-11 Revision Conference in Tokyo, Japan. In addition, a wide range of countries attended the Tokyo Revision Conference including: Albania; Algeria; Argentina; Australia; Brazil; Cambodia; Canada; China; Denmark; Egypt; Ethiopia; Finland; India; Indonesia; Iran; Japan; Kenya; Korea; Kuwait; Malaysia; Mexico; Mozambique; Myanmar; Namibia; Nepal; Netherlands; Philippines; Republic of Korea; Russian Federation; Rwanda; Slovakia; Sri Lanka; Sweden; Tanzania; Thailand; Turkmenistan; Uganda; United Kingdom; and the United States of America." The full report is available on the WHO Website: http://who.int/classifications/network/meeting2016/ICD- 11RevisionConferenceReportTokyo.pdf?ua=1.

[67] Perronne C (2014) Lyme and associated tick-borne diseases: Global challenges of Lyme disease. Front. Cell. Infect. Microbiol. 4:74

Stanek G and Reiter M (2011) The expanding Lyme Borrelia complex – Clinical significance of genomic species? Clin Microbiol Infect;17(4):487-93. http://www.ncbi.nlm.nih.gov/pubmed/21414082

Bibliography

1990 syphilis case definition. https://wwwn.cdc.gov/nndss/conditions/syphilis/case-definition/1990/. Accessed January 29, 2017.

1996 syphilis case definition. https://wwwn.cdc.gov/nndss/conditions/syphilis/case-definition/1996/. Accessed January 29, 2017.

2014 syphilis case definition. https://wwwn.cdc.gov/nndss/conditions/syphilis/case-definition/2014/. Accessed January 29, 2017.

A global brief on vector-borne diseases, World Health Organization No. WHO/DCO/WHD/2014.1, (2014). http://apps.who.int/iris/bitstream/10665/111008/1/WHO_DCO_WHD_2014.1_eng.pdf. Accessed February 15, 2017.

A Timeline of HIV/AIDS. https://www.aids.gov/hiv-aids-basics/hiv-aids-101/aids-timeline/. Accessed January 29, 2017.

Aasly J, Nilsen G. Cerebral atrophy in Lyme disease. *Neuroradiology*. 1990;32(3):252-252. doi:10.1007/bf00589125. [PubMed]

Abele DC, Anders KH, Chandler FW. Benign lymphocytic infiltration (Jessner-Kanof): another manifestation of borreliosis? *J Am Acad Dermatol*. 1989;21(4 Pt 1):795-7. https://www.ncbi.nlm.nih.gov/pubmed/2808795

Aberer E, Schmidt BL, Breier F, Kinaciyan T, Luger A. Amplification of DNA of Borrelia burgdorferi in urine samples of patients with granuloma annulare and lichen sclerosus et atrophicus. 1999;135(2):210-2. https://www.ncbi.nlm.nih.gov/pubmed/10052416

Ackermann R, Gollmer E, Rehse-Küpper B. [Progressive Borrelia encephalomyelitis. Chronic manifestation of erythema chronicum migrans disease of the nervous system] [in German]. *DMW - Deutsche Medizinische Wochenschrift*. 1985;110(26):1039–1042. doi:10.1055/s-2008-1068956. [PubMed]

Adamaszek M, Heinrich A, Rang A, Langner S, Khaw AV. Cerebral sinuvenous thrombosis associated with Lyme neuroborreliosis. *Journal of Neurology*. 2009;257(3):481–483. doi:10.1007/s00415-009-5397-7.

Adrion ER, Aucott J, Lemke KW, Weiner JP. Health care costs, utilization and patterns of care following Lyme disease. *PLOS ONE*. 2015;10(2):e0116767. doi:10.1371/journal.pone.0116767.

Africa Fact Sheet - Main Economic Indicators, United Nations Office of the Special Advisor on Africa (OSAA) and the NEPAD-OECD Africa Investment Initiative, (2005). https://www.oecd.org/investment/investmentfordevelopment/47452483.pdf. Accessed February 15, 2017.

Alban PS, Nelson DR, Johnson PW. Serum-starvation-induced changes in protein synthesis and morphology of Borrelia burgdorferi. *Microbiology*. 2000;146(1):119-127. doi:10.1099/00221287-146-1-119.

Allen HB, Morales D. Alzheimers disease: A novel hypothesis integrating spirochetes, biofilm, and the immune system. *Journal of Neuroinfectious Diseases*. 2016;07(01). doi:10.4172/2314-7326.1000200.

Almeida OP, Lautenschlager NT. Dementia associated with infectious diseases. *International Psychogeriatrics*. 2005;17(S1):S65. doi:10.1017/s104161020500195x. [PubMed]

Almoussa M1, Goertzen A1, Fauser B1, Zimmermann CW1. Stroke as an Unusual First Presentation of Lyme Disease. Case Rep Neurol Med. 2015; 2015:389081. doi: 10.1155/2015/389081.

Altizer S, Ostfeld RS, Johnson PTJ, Kutz S, Harvell CD. Climate change and infectious diseases: From evidence to a predictive framework. *Science*. 2013;341(6145):514-519. doi:10.1126/science.1239401.

Arboviral diseases, Neuroinvasive and Non-neuroinvasive. https://wwwn.cdc.gov/nndss/conditions/arboviral-diseases-neuroinvasive-and-non-neuroinvasive/case-definition/2004. Accessed January 29, 2017.

Arnež M, Ružić-Sabljić E. Borrelial Lymphocytoma in Children. *Pediatr Infect Dis J*. 2015;34(12):1319-22.

Asbrink E, Brehmer-Andersson E, Hovmark A. Acrodermatitis chronica atrophicans--a spirochetosis. Clinical and histopathological picture based on 32 patients; course and relationship to erythema chronicum migrans Afzelius. *Am J Dermatopathol*. 1986;8(3):209-19.
https://www.ncbi.nlm.nih.gov/pubmed/3728879

Asbrink E, Hovmark A. Lyme borreliosis: aspects of tick-borne Borrelia burgdorferi infection from a dermatologic viewpoint. Semin Dermatol. 1990;9(4):277-91. Review.
https://www.ncbi.nlm.nih.gov/pubmed/2285572

Askling J, Dixon W. The safety of anti-tumour necrosis factor therapy in rheumatoid arthritis. *Current Opinion in Rheumatology*. 2008;20(2):138-144. doi:10.1097/bor.0b013e3282f4b392.

Bacino L, Gazzarata M, Siri G, Cordone S, Bellotti P. [Complete atrioventricular block as the first clinical manifestation of a tick bite (Lyme disease)] [in Italian]. *Giornale italiano di cardiologia (2006)*. 2011;12(3):214-6. https://www.ncbi.nlm.nih.gov/pubmed/21560478. Accessed February 13, 2017.

Back T, Grünig S, Winter Y, et al. Neuroborreliosis-associated cerebral vasculitis: Long-term outcome and health-related quality of life. *Journal of Neurology*. 2013;260(6):1569-1575. doi:10.1007/s00415-013-6831-4.

Bahrain H, Laureno R, Krishnan J, Aggarwal A, Malkovska V. Lyme disease mimicking central nervous system lymphoma. *Cancer Investigation*. 2007;25(5):336-339. doi:10.1080/07357900701357977.

Bale JF, Murph JR. Congenital infections and the nervous system. *Pediatric Clinics of North America*. 1992;39(4):669-690. doi:10.1016/s0031-3955(16)38370-5.

Baldari U, Cattonar P, Nobile C, Celli B, Righini MG, Trevisan G. Infantile acrodermatitis of Gianotti-Crosti and Lyme borreliosis. *Acta Derm Venereol*. 1996;76(3):242-3.
https://www.ncbi.nlm.nih.gov/pubmed/8800310

Baltimore Afro-American - Google news archive search.
https://news.google.com/newspapers?nid=2205&dat=19821218&id=7PkmAAAAIBAJ&sjid=MAMGAAAAIBAJ&pg=1370,4750215. Accessed January 29, 2017.

Batinac T, Petranovic D, Zamolo G, Ruzic A. Lyme borreliosis and multiple sclerosis are associated with primary effusion lymphoma. *Medical Hypotheses*. 2007;69(1):117-119. doi:10.1016/j.mehy.2006.11.015.

Beermann C. Lipoproteins from Borrelia burgdorferi applied in liposomes and presented by Dendritic cells induce CD8+ t-lymphocytes in vitro. *Cellular Immunology*. 2000;201(2):124-131. http://www.sciencedirect.com/science/article/pii/S000887490091640X. Accessed January 29, 2017.

Bendig JWA, Ogilvie D. Severe encephalopathy associated with lyme disease. *The Lancet*. 1987;329(8534):681-682. doi:10.1016/s0140-6736(87)90440-5.

Benedix F, Weide B, Broekaert S, et al. Early disseminated borreliosis with multiple erythema migrans and elevated liver enzymes: case report and literature review. *Acta Derm Venereol*. 2007;87(5):418-421. doi:10.2340/00015555-0267.

Bensch J, Olcén P, Hagberg L. Destructive chronic Borelia Meningoencephalitis in a child untreated for 15 years. *Scandinavian Journal of Infectious Diseases*. 1987;19(6):697-700. doi:10.3109/00365548709117207. [PubMed]

Berndtson K. Review of evidence for immune evasion and persistent infection in Lyme | IJGM. *International Journal of General Medicine*. 2013; Volume 6:291-306. doi:10.2147/IJGM.S44114. http://dx.doi.org/10.2147/IJGM.S44114. Accessed February 19, 2017.

Bertrand E, Szpak GM, Piłkowska E, et al. Central nervous system infection caused by Borrelia burgdorferi. Clinico-pathological correlation of three post-mortem cases. *Folia neuropathologica*. 1999;37(1):43-51. https://www.ncbi.nlm.nih.gov/pubmed/10337063. Accessed February 27, 2017. [PubMed]

Błaut-Jurkowska J1, Olszowska M1, Kaźnica-Wiatr M1, Podolec P1. [Lyme carditis]. Pol Merkur Lekarski. 2015 Aug;39(230):111-5.

Blažina K1, Miletić V, Relja M, Bažadona D. Cerebral sinuvenous thrombosis: a rare complication of Lyme neuroborreliosis. Wien Klin Wochenschr. 2015 Jan;127(1-2):65-7. doi: 10.1007/s00508-014-0622-5.

Buechner SA, Winkelmann RK, Lautenschlager S, Gilli L, Rufli T. Localized scleroderma associated with Borrelia burgdorferi infection. Clinical, histologic, and immunohistochemical observations. *J Am Acad Dermatol*. 1993;29(2 Pt 1):190-6. https://www.ncbi.nlm.nih.gov/pubmed/8335737

Bockenstedt LK, Gonzalez DG, Haberman AM, Belperron AA. Spirochete antigens persist near cartilage after murine Lyme borreliosis therapy. *The Journal of Clinical Investigation*. 2012;122(7):2652-2660. doi:10.1172/JCI58813. http://www.jci.org/articles/view/58813. Accessed January 29, 2017.

Bogsrud TV, Odegaard B. [Tick-borne borreliosis. A case of chronic meningoencephalitis caused by Borrelia burgdorferi] [in Norwegian]. *Tidsskrift for den Norske laegeforening : tidsskrift for praktisk medicin, ny raekke*. 1987;107(1):25-7. https://www.ncbi.nlm.nih.gov/pubmed/3824285. Accessed February 27, 2017. [PubMed]

Borgermans L, Perronne C, Balicer R, Polasek O, Obsomer V. Lyme disease: Time for a new approach? *BMJ*. December 2015:h6520. doi:10.1136/bmj.h6520.

Braun J, Laitko S, Treharne J, et al. Chlamydia pneumoniae--a new causative agent of reactive arthritis and undifferentiated oligoarthritis. *Annals of the Rheumatic Diseases*. 1994;53(2):100-105. doi:10.1136/ard.53.2.100. http://ard.bmj.com/content/53/2/100. Accessed January 29, 2017.

Brogan GX, Homan CS, Vicellio P. The enlarging clinical spectrum of lyme disease: Lyme cerebral vasculitis, a new disease entity. *Annals of Emergency Medicine*. 1990;19(5):572-576. doi:10.1016/s0196-0644(05)83017-3. [PubMed]

Brorson Ø, Brorson S, Henriksen T, Skogen PR, Schoyen R. Association between multiple sclerosis and cystic structures in Cerebrospinal fluid. *Infection*. 2001;29(6):315-319. doi:10.1007/s15010-001-9144-y.

Brorson Ø, Brorson S. An in vitro study of the susceptibility of mobile and cystic forms of Borrelia burgdorferi to hydroxychloroquine. *International Microbiology*. 2002;5(1):25-31. doi:10.1007/s10123-002-0055-2.

Brorson Ø, Brorson S-H. A rapid method for generating cystic forms of Borrelia burgdorferi, and their reversal to mobile spirochetes. *APMIS*. 1998;106(7-12):1131-1141. doi:10.1111/j.1699-0463.1998.tb00269.x.

Brzostek T. [Human granulocytic ehrlichiosis co-incident with Lyme borreliosis in pregnant woman--a case study] [in Polish]. *Przegl Epidemiol*. 2004;58(2):289-94.

Bu XL, Yao XQ, Jiao SS, et al. A study on the association between infectious burden and Alzheimer's disease. *European Journal of Neurology*. 2014;22(12):1519-1525. doi:10.1111/ene.12477.

Buechner SA, Winkelmann RK, Lautenschlager S, Gilli L, Rufli T. Localized scleroderma associated with Borrelia burgdorferi infection. Clinical, histologic, and immunohistochemical observations. *J Am Acad Dermatol*. 1993;29(2 Pt 1):190-6. https://www.ncbi.nlm.nih.gov/pubmed/8335737

Burakgazi AZ. Lyme disease -induced polyradiculopathy mimicking amyotrophic lateral sclerosis. *International Journal of Neuroscience*. 2014;124(11):859-862. doi:10.3109/00207454.2013.879582.

Burgdorfer W. Discovery of the Lyme disease spirochete and its relation to tick vectors. *The Yale journal of biology and medicine*. 1984;57(4):515-20. https://www.ncbi.nlm.nih.gov/pubmed/6516454. Accessed February 19, 2017.

Burgdorfer W. Lyme borreliosis: Ten years after discovery of the etiologic agent, Borrelia burgdorferi. *Infection*. 1991;19(4):257-262. doi:10.1007/bf01644963.

Busch U, Hizo-Teufel C, Böhmer R, Fingerle V, Rössler D, Wilske B, Preac-Mursic V. Borrelia burgdorferi sensu lato strains isolated from cutaneous Lyme borreliosis biopsies differentiated by pulsed-field gel electrophoresis. *Scand J Infect Dis*. 1996;28(6):583-9.
https://www.ncbi.nlm.nih.gov/pubmed/9060061

Buzzard EF. The treatment of disseminated sclerosis: a suggestion. *The Lancet*. 1911;177(4559):98. doi:10.1016/s0140-6736(01)60085-0.

Cameron DJ, Johnson LB, Maloney EL. Evidence assessments and guideline recommendations in Lyme disease: The clinical management of known tick bites, erythema migrans rashes and persistent disease. *Expert Review of Anti-infective Therapy*. 2014;12(9):1103-1135. doi:10.1586/14787210.2014.940900.

Carlomagno G, Luksa V, Candussi G, Rizzi G, Trevisan G. Lyme Borrelia positive serology associated with spontaneous abortion in an endemic Italian area. *Acta Europaea fertilitatis*. 1988;19(5):279-81. https://www.ncbi.nlm.nih.gov/pubmed/3252658. Accessed February 24, 2017.

Case definitions for public health surveillance. https://wonder.cdc.gov/wonder/prevguid/m0025629/m0025629.asp. Accessed January 29, 2017.

Cassarino DS, Quezado MM, Ghatak NR, Duray PH. Lyme-associated parkinsonism: A neuropathologic case study and review of the literature. *Archives of pathology & laboratory medicine*. 2003;127(9):1204-6. https://www.ncbi.nlm.nih.gov/pubmed/12946221. Accessed February 24, 2017. [PubMed]

CDC. CDC provides estimate of Americans diagnosed with Lyme disease each year. https://www.cdc.gov/media/releases/2013/p0819-lyme-disease.html. Accessed January 29, 2017.

CDC. Current trends Lyme disease surveillance -- United States, 1989 - 1990. https://www.cdc.gov/mmwr/preview/mmwrhtml/00014526.htm. Accessed January 29, 2017.

CDC. Lyme disease. https://www.cdc.gov/lyme/index.html. Accessed January 29, 2017.

CDC. MMWR: Summary of Notifiable infectious diseases. https://www.cdc.gov/mmwr/mmwr_nd/index.html. Accessed January 29, 2017.

CDC. Resources for health professionals. http://www.cdc.gov/parasites/babesiosis/health_professionals/. Accessed January 30, 2017.

CDC. Signs and symptoms (Q Fever). https://www.cdc.gov/qfever/symptoms/index.html. Accessed January 29, 2017.

CDC. Signs and symptoms of untreated Lyme disease. https://www.cdc.gov/lyme/signs_symptoms/index.html. Accessed January 29, 2017.

CDC. Treatment for valley fever (coccidioidomycosis). https://www.cdc.gov/fungal/diseases/coccidioidomycosis/treatment.html. Accessed January 29, 2017.

Chary-Valckenaere I. Ultrastructural demonstration of intracellular localization of Borrelia burgdorferi in Lyme arthritis. *Rheumatology*. 1998;37(4):468-470. doi:10.1093/rheumatology/37.4.468.

Chavanet P, Pillon D, Lancon JP, Waldner-Combernoux A, Maringe E, Portier H. Granulomatous hepatitis associated with lyme disease. *The Lancet*. 1987;330(8559):623-624. doi:10.1016/s0140-6736(87)93009-1.

Christova I, Komitova R. Clinical and epidemiological features of Lyme borreliosis in Bulgaria. *Wien Klin Wochenschr*. 2004;116(1-2):42-6. https://www.ncbi.nlm.nih.gov/pubmed/15030123

Cimmino MA, Trevisan G. Lyme arthritis presenting as adult onset still's disease. *Clinical and experimental rheumatology*. 1989;7(3):305-8. https://www.ncbi.nlm.nih.gov/pubmed/2667831. Accessed February 26, 2017.

Cimperman J, Maraspin V, Lotric-Furlan S, Ruzić-Sabljić E, Avsic-Zupanc T, Strle F. Diffuse reversible alopecia in patients with Lyme meningitis and tick-borne encephalitis. *Wiener klinische Wochenschrift*. 1999;10;111(22-23):976-72000;111:976-7. https://www.ncbi.nlm.nih.gov/pubmed/10666812. Accessed February 13, 2017.

Climate change indicators: Lyme disease. United States Environmental Protection Agency. https://www.epa.gov/climate-indicators/climate-change-indicators-lyme-disease. Accessed February 15, 2017.

Clinckaert C, Bidgoli S, Verbeet T, et al. Peroperative cardiogenic shock suggesting acute coronary syndrome as initial manifestation of Lyme carditis. *Journal of Clinical Anesthesia*. 2016;35:430-433. doi:10.1016/j.jclinane.2016.08.005.

Coblyn JS, Taylor P. Treatment of chronic Lyme arthritis with Hydroxychloroquine. *Arthritis & Rheumatism*. 1981;24(12):1567-1569. doi:10.1002/art.1780241217.

Colli C, Leinweber B, Müllegger R, Chott A, Kerl H, Cerroni L. Borrelia burgdorferi-associated lymphocytoma cutis: clinicopathologic, immunophenotypic, and molecular study of 106 cases. *J Cutan Pathol*. 2004;31(3):232-40. https://www.ncbi.nlm.nih.gov/pubmed/14984575

Cook M, Puri B. Commercial test kits for detection of Lyme borreliosis: A meta-analysis of test accuracy. *International Journal of General Medicine*. 2016;Volume 9:427-440. doi:10.2147/ijgm.s122313.

Coulter P, Lema C, Flayhart D, et al. Two-year evaluation of Borrelia burgdorferi culture and supplemental tests for definitive diagnosis of Lyme disease. *Journal of clinical microbiology.* 2005;43(10):5080-4. https://www.ncbi.nlm.nih.gov/pubmed/16207966. Accessed February 15, 2017.

Coyle PK, Deng Z, Schutzer SE, et al. Detection of Borrelia burgdorferi antigens in cerebrospinal fluid. *Neurology.* 1993;43(6):1093-1093. doi:10.1212/wnl.43.6.1093.

Coyle PK, Schutzer SE, Deng Z, et al. Detection of Borrelia burgdorferi-specific antigen in antibody-negative cerebrospinal fluid in neurologic Lyme disease. *Neurology.* 1995;45(11):2010-2015. doi:10.1212/wnl.45.11.2010.

Coyle PK. Borrelia burgdorferi antibodies in multiple sclerosis patients. *Neurology.* 1989;39(6):760-760. doi:10.1212/wnl.39.6.760.

Créange A. [Clinical manifestations and epidemiological aspects leading to a diagnosis of Lyme borreliosis: Neurological and psychiatric manifestations in the course of Lyme borreliosis] [in French]. *Medecine et maladies infectieuses.* 2007;37:532-9. https://www.ncbi.nlm.nih.gov/pubmed/17368785. Accessed February 23, 2017.

Cuisset T, Hamilos M, Vanderheyden M. Coronary aneurysm in Lyme disease: Treatment by covered stent. *International Journal of Cardiology.* 2008;128(2):e72-e73. doi:10.1016/j.ijcard.2007.04.163.

Cutler SJ, Rudenko N, Golovchenko M, et al. Diagnosing Borreliosis. *Vector-Borne and Zoonotic Diseases.* 2017;17(1):2-11. doi:10.1089/vbz.2016.1962.

Czyrny M, Jura E, Seniów J, Barańska M, Wilske B, Członkowska A. [Severe meningoencephalitis in Borrelia burgdorferi infection] [in Polish]. *Neurologia i neurochirurgia polska.* 1998;32(2):387-93. https://www.ncbi.nlm.nih.gov/pubmed/9760557. Accessed February 27, 2017. [PubMed]

Dalal MA, Wehrle R, Beitinger PA, Wetter TC. Lyme borreliosis presenting as hypersomnia. *Somnologie - Schlafforschung und Schlafmedizin.* 2010;14(1):67-69. doi:10.1007/s11818-010-0455-z.

Dattwyler RJ, Volkman DJ, Luft BJ, Halperin JJ, Thomas J, Golightly MG. Seronegative Lyme Disease. Dissociation of T- and B-Lymphocyte Responses to Borrelia burgdorferi. *N Engl J Med* 1988;319:1441-6. DOI: 10.1056/NEJM198812013192203

De Cauwer H, Declerck S, De Smet J, et al. Motor neuron disease features in a patient with neuroborreliosis and a cervical anterior horn lesion. *Acta Clinica Belgica.* 2009;64(3):225-227. doi:10.1179/acb.2009.039. [PubMed]

Defer G, Levy R, Brugiéres P, Postic D, Degos JD. Lyme disease presenting as a stroke in the vertebrobasilar territory: MRI. *Neuroradiology.* 1993;35(7):529-31. https://www.ncbi.nlm.nih.gov/pubmed/8232882. Accessed February 26, 2017. [PubMed]

DellaSala DA, Middelveen M, Liegner KB, Luche-Thayer J. Lyme disease epidemic increasing globally due to climate change and human activities. *The Encyclopedia of the Anthropocene.* in press.

Dernedde S, Piper C, Kühl U, et al. [The Lyme carditis as a rare differential diagnosis to an anterior myocardial infarction] [in German]. *Zeitschrift für Kardiologie*. 2002;91(12):1053-1060. doi:10.1007/s00392-002-0873-4.

Diatta G, Duplantier J-M, Granjon L, et al. Borrelia infection in small mammals in west Africa and its relationship with tick occurrence inside burrows. *Acta Tropica*. 2015;152:131-140. doi:10.1016/j.actatropica.2015.08.016.

Dinerman H. Lyme disease associated with Fibromyalgia. *Annals of Internal Medicine*. 1992;117(4):281. doi:10.7326/0003-4819-117-4-281.

Diringer MN, Halperin JJ, Dattwyler RJ. Lyme meningoencephalitis: Report of a severe, penicillin-resistant case. *Arthritis and rheumatism*. 1987;30(6):705-8. https://www.ncbi.nlm.nih.gov/pubmed/3649235. Accessed February 27, 2017. [PubMed]

Donta ST. Macrolide therapy of chronic Lyme disease. *Med SCI Monit*. 2003;2003(9(11)):136-142. http://lymeaware.free.fr/lyme/Diagnostiques/References/2011_0187_0004_TSTMNY_macrolide_therapy_lyme_disease.pdf. Accessed January 29, 2017.

Dörner T, Jacobi AM, Lipsky PE. B cells in autoimmunity. *Arthritis Research & Therapy*. 2009;11(5):247. doi:10.1186/ar2780.

Dorward DW, Fischer ER, Brooks DM. Invasion and Cytopathic killing of human lymphocytes by Spirochetes causing Lyme disease. *Clinical Infectious Diseases*. 1997;25(s1):S2-S8. doi:10.1086/516169.

Drenckhahn A, Spors B, Knierim E. Acute isolated partial oculomotor nerve palsy due to Lyme neuroborreliosis in a 5 year old girl. *Eur J Paediatr Neurol EJPN Off J Eur Paediatr Neurol Soc*. 2016;20(6):977-979. doi:10.1016/j.ejpn.2016.05.022

Drouet A, Meyer X, Guilloton L, et al. [Acute severe leukoencephalitis with posterior lesions due to Borrelia burgdorferi infection] [in French]. *Presse medicale (Paris, France : 1983)*. 2003;32(34):1607-9. https://www.ncbi.nlm.nih.gov/pubmed/14576583. Accessed February 27, 2017. [PubMed]

Dupuis M. [Multiple neurologic manifestations of Borrelia burgdorferi infection] [in French]. *Revue neurologique*. 1988;144(12):765-75. https://www.ncbi.nlm.nih.gov/pubmed/3070690. Accessed March 1, 2017. [PubMed]

Duray PH, Steere AC. Clinical pathologic correlations of Lyme disease by stage. *Annals of the New York Academy of Sciences*. 1988;539(1 Lyme Disease):65-79. doi:10.1111/j.1749-6632.1988.tb31839.x. [PubMed]

Duray PH, Steere AC. The spectrum of organ and systems pathology in human lyme disease. *Zentralblatt für Bakteriologie, Mikrobiologie und Hygiene. Series A: Medical Microbiology, Infectious Diseases, Virology, Parasitology*. 1986;263(1-2):169-178. doi:10.1016/s0176-6724(86)80120-1. [PubMed]

Duray PH. Histopathology of clinical phases of human Lyme disease. *Rheumatic diseases clinics of North America*. 1989;15(4):691-710. https://www.ncbi.nlm.nih.gov/pubmed/2685926. Accessed February 27, 2017. [PubMed]

Duray PH. The surgical pathology of human Lyme disease. *The American Journal of Surgical Pathology*. 1987;11(Supplement1):47-60. doi:10.1097/00000478-198700111-00005. [PubMed]

Dworkin MS, Schwan TG, Anderson DE, Borchardt SM. Tick-borne Relapsing fever. *Infectious Disease Clinics of North America*. 2008;22(3):449-468. doi:10.1016/j.idc.2008.03.006. https://uic.pure.elsevier.com/en/publications/tick-borne-relapsing-fever. Accessed February 19, 2017.

Eisendle K, Grabner T, Zelger B. Morphoea: a manifestation of infection with Borrelia species? *Br J Dermatol*. 2007;157(6):1189-98. DOI: 10.1111/j.1365-2133.2007.08235.x

Embers ME, Barthold SW, Borda JT, et al. Persistence of Borrelia burgdorferi in Rhesus Macaques following antibiotic treatment of disseminated infection. *PLoS ONE*. 2012;7(1):e29914. doi:10.1371/journal.pone.0029914.

European Centre for Disease Prevention and Control. Meeting Report. Paper presented at: Second expert consultation on tick-borne diseases with emphasis on Lyme borreliosis and tick-borne encephalitis; November 22, 2011; Stockholm, Sweden. http://ecdc.europa.eu/en/publications/Publications/Tick-borne-diseases-meeting-report.pdf. Accessed February 15, 2017.

Fallon B, Nields JA. Lyme disease: A neuropsychiatric illness. *American Journal of Psychiatry*. 1994;151(11):1571-1583. doi:10.1176/ajp.151.11.1571. [PubMed]

Fallon BA, Das S, Plutchok JJ, Tager F, Liegner K, Van Heertum R. Functional brain imaging and Neuropsychological testing in Lyme disease. *Clinical Infectious Diseases*. 1997;25(s1):S57-S63. doi:10.1086/516175.

Fallon BA, Kochevar JM, Gaito A, Nields JA. The underdiagnosis of neuropsychiatric Lyme disease in children and adults. *Psychiatric Clinics of North America*. 1998;21(3):693-703. doi:10.1016/s0193-953x(05)70032-0.

Fallon BA, Schwartzberg M, Bransfield R, et al. Late-stage neuropsychiatric Lyme Borreliosis. *Psychosomatics*. 1995;36(3):295-300. doi:10.1016/s0033-3182(95)71669-3.

Fallon BA. Regional cerebral blood flow and cognitive deficits in chronic Lyme disease. *Journal of Neuropsychiatry*. 2003;15(3):326-332. doi:10.1176/appi.neuropsych.15.3.326.

Federlin K, Becker H. [Borrelia infection and systemic lupus erythematosus] [in German]. *Immunitat und Infektion*. 1989;17(6):195-8. https://www.ncbi.nlm.nih.gov/pubmed/2693342. Accessed February 24, 2017.

Fénelon G, Chaine P, Lèche J, Guillard A. [Isolated meningoencephalitis in Lyme disease] [in French]. *Annales de medecine interne*. 1987;138(2):149-50. https://www.ncbi.nlm.nih.gov/pubmed/3579101. Accessed February 27, 2017. [PubMed]

Feng J, Shi W, Zhang S, Sullivan D, Auwaerter PG, Zhang Y. A drug combination screen identifies drugs active against Amoxicillin-Induced round bodies of in vitro Borrelia burgdorferi Persisters from an FDA drug library. *Frontiers in Microbiology*. 2016;7. doi:10.3389/fmicb.2016.00743.

Feng J, Shi W, Zhang S, Zhang Y. Persister mechanisms in Borrelia burgdorferi: Implications for improved intervention. *Emerging Microbes & Infections*. 2015;4(8):e51. doi:10.1038/emi.2015.51.

Feng J, Weitner M, Shi W, Zhang S, Zhang Y. Eradication of Biofilm-Like Microcolony structures of Borrelia burgdorferi by Daunomycin and Daptomycin but not Mitomycin C in combination with Doxycycline and Cefuroxime. *Frontiers in Microbiology*. 2016;7. doi:10.3389/fmicb.2016.00062.

Feng J, Zhang S, Shi W, Zhang Y. Ceftriaxone pulse Dosing fails to eradicate Biofilm-Like Microcolony B. Burgdorferi Persisters which are sterilized by Daptomycin/ Doxycycline/Cefuroxime without pulse Dosing. *Frontiers in Microbiology*. 2016;7. doi:10.3389/fmicb.2016.01744.

Ferroir JP, Reignier A, Nicolle MH, Guillard A. [Meningoradiculoencephalitis in Lyme disease. A case with major regressive mental disorders] [in French]. *Presse medicale (Paris, France : 1983)*. 1988;17(14). https://www.ncbi.nlm.nih.gov/pubmed/2966957. Accessed February 27, 2017. [PubMed]

Fikrig E, Narasimhan S. Borrelia burgdorferi-Traveling incognito? *Microbes and Infection*. 2006;8(5):1390-1399. doi:10.1016/j.micinf.2005.12.022.

Fiscal Year 2016, Centers for Disease Control and Prevention, Justification of Estimates for Appropriation Committees, U.S. Department of Health and Human Services, pt Performance measure for Long Term Objective: Protect Americans from Infectious Diseases—Vector-borne., at 417 (2015). https://www.cdc.gov/budget/documents/fy2016/fy-2016-cdc-congressional-justification.pdf. Accessed February 15, 2017.

Florens N, Lemoine S, Guebre-Egziabher F, et al. Chronic Lyme borreliosis associated with minimal change glomerular disease: a case report. *BMC Nephrol*. 2017;18(1). doi:10.1186/s12882-017-0462-4.

Forrester JD, Mead P. Third-Degree heart block associated with Lyme Carditis: Review of published cases. *Clinical Infectious Diseases*. 2014;59(7):996-1000. doi:10.1093/cid/ciu411.

Furr PM, Taylor-Robinson D, Webster AD. Mycoplasmas and ureaplasmas in patients with hypogammaglobulinaemia and their role in arthritis: Microbiological observations over twenty years. *Annals of the Rheumatic Diseases*. 1994;53(3):183-187. doi:10.1136/ard.53.3.183.

Gamble JL, Ebi KL, Grambsch AE, Sussman FG, Wilbanks TJ. Analyses of the Effects of Global Change on Human Health and Welfare and Human Systems, U.S. Environmental Protection Agency Report by the U.S. Climate Change Science Program and the Subcommittee on Global Change Research No. Synthesis and Assessment Product 4.6, (2008). https://downloads.globalchange.gov/sap/sap4-6/sap4-6-final-report-all.pdf. Accessed February 18, 2017.

Garbe C, Stein H, Dienemann D, Orfanos CE. Borrelia burgdorferi—associated cutaneous B cell lymphoma: Clinical and immunohistologic characterization of four cases. *Journal of the American Academy of Dermatology*. 1991;24(4):584-590. doi:10.1016/0190-9622(91)70088-j.

García-Moncó JC, Jornet M, Villar F, Benach JL, Espejo G, Berciano JA. [Multiple sclerosis or Lyme disease? A diagnosis problem of exclusion] [in Spanish]. *Medicina clinica*. 1990;94(18):685-8. https://www.ncbi.nlm.nih.gov/pubmed/2388492. Accessed February 26, 2017.

Garcia-Moncó JC, Wheeler CM, Benach JL, et al. Reactivity of neuroborreliosis patients (Lyme disease) to cardiolipin and gangliosides. *Journal of the Neurological Sciences*. 1993;117(1-2):206-214. doi:10.1016/0022-510x(93)90175-x.

Gardner T. Lyme disease. In: Remington JS, Klein JO, eds. *Infectious Diseases of the Fetus and Newborn*. 5th ed. Philadelphia: Saunders; 1995:447-528chap 11.

Gardner T. Lyme disease. In: Remington JS, Klein JO. *Infectious diseases of the fetus and newborn infant*. 4th ed. Philadelphia: W B Saunders Co; December 13, 1994.

Gardner T. Lyme disease: 66 Pregnancies complicated by Lyme Borreliosis. In: Remington JS, Klein JO, eds. *Clinical Infectious Diseases*. 5th ed. Philadelphia: Oxford University Press (OUP); August 2001.

Garon CF, Dorward DW, Corwin MD. Structural features of Borrelia burgdorferi the Lyme disease spirochete: Silver staining for nucleic acids. *Scanning Microsc Suppl*. 1989;3:109-15. http://science.report/pub/33227357. Accessed January 29, 2017.

Gasser R, Watzinger N, Eber B, et al. Coronary artery aneurysm in two patients with long-standing Lyme borreliosis. *The Lancet*. 1994;344(8932):1300-1301. doi:10.1016/s0140-6736(94)90789-7.

Glatz M, Resinger A, Semmelweis K, Ambros-Rudolph CM, Müllegger RR. Clinical spectrum of skin manifestations of Lyme borreliosis in 204 children in Austria. *Acta Derm Venereol*. 2015;95(5):565-71. doi: 10.2340/00015555-2000.

Gérard P, Canaple S, Rosa A. [Meningopapillitis disclosing Lyme disease] [in French]. *Revue neurologique*. 1996;152:476-8. https://www.ncbi.nlm.nih.gov/pubmed/8944247. Accessed February 26, 2017.

Goebel KM, Krause A, Neurath F. Acquired transient autoimmune reactions in Lyme arthritis: Correlation between rheumatoid factor and disease activity. *Scandinavian Journal of Rheumatology*. 1988;17(sup75):314-317. doi:10.3109/03009748809096784.

Goellner MH. Hepatitis due to recurrent Lyme disease. *Annals of Internal Medicine*. 1988;108(5):707. doi:10.7326/0003-4819-108-5-707.

Goldenberg RL, Thompson C. The infectious origins of stillbirth. *American Journal of Obstetrics and Gynecology*. 2003;189(3):861-873. doi:10.1067/s0002-9378(03)00470-8.

Golubić D, Vinković T, Turk D, Hranilović J, Slugan I. [Ocular manifestations of Lyme borreliosis in northwest Croatia]. *Lijec Vjesn*. 2004;126(5-6):124-128.

Gordillo-Pérez G, Torres J, Solórzano-Santos F, de Martino S, Lipsker D, Velázquez E, Ramon G, Onofre M, Jaulhac B. Borrelia burgdorferi infection and cutaneous Lyme disease, Mexico. *Emerg Infect Dis*. 2007;13(10):1556-8. DOI: 10.3201/eid1310.060630

Grading of Recommendations Assessment, Development and Evaluation Working Group. Welcome to the GRADE working group. GRADE. https://www.gradeworkinggroup.org/. Accessed February 18, 2017.

Grankvist A, Andersson P, Mattsson M, et al. Infections with the tick-borne bacterium "Candidatus Neoehrlichia mikurensis" mimic Noninfectious conditions in patients with B cell malignancies or autoimmune diseases. *Clinical Infectious Diseases*. 2014;58(12):1716-1722. doi:10.1093/cid/ciu189.

Gratz NG. *The vector-borne human infections of europe - their distribution and burden on public health*. Switzerland: World Health Organization; 2004. http://www.euro.who.int/_data/assets/pdf_file/0008/98765/e82481.pdf. Accessed February 18, 2017.

Greco T, Conti-Kelly A. Antiphospholipid antibodies in patients with purported "chronic Lyme disease." *Lupus*. 2011;20(13):1372-1377. doi:10.1177/0961203311414098.

Gruntar I, Malovrh T, Murgia R, Cinco M. Conversion of Borrelia garinii cystic forms to motile spirochetes in vivoNote. *APMIS*. 2001;109(5):383-388. doi:10.1034/j.1600-0463.2001.090507.x.

Gubertini N, Bonin S, Trevisan G. Lichen sclerosus et atrophicans, scleroderma en coup de sabre and Lyme borreliosis. *Dermatol Reports*. 2011;28;3(2):e27. doi: 10.4081/dr.2011.e27.

Guenther F, Bode C, Faber T. [Reversible complete heart block by re-infection with Borrelia burgdorferi with negative IgM-antibodies] [in German]. *Deutsche medizinische Wochenschrift (1946)*. 2008;134:23-6. https://www.ncbi.nlm.nih.gov/pubmed/19090448. Accessed February 13, 2017.

Gustafson JM, Burgess EC, Wachal MD, Steinberg H. Intrauterine transmission of Borrelia burgdorferi in dogs. *American Journal of Veterinary Research*. 1993;54(6):882-890. http://europepmc.org/abstract/med/8323057. Accessed February 13, 2017.

Habek M1, Mubrin Z, Brinar VV. Avellis syndrome due to borreliosis. Eur J Neurol. 2007 Jan;14(1):112-4.

Haarala M, Kiiholma P, Nurmi M, Uksila J, Alanen A. The role of *Borrelia burgdorferi* in interstitial Cystitis. *European Urology*. 2000;37(4):395-399. doi:10.1159/000020184.

Halperin JJ, Kaplan GP, Brazinsky S, et al. Immunologic reactivity against Borrelia burgdorferi in patients with motor neuron disease. *Archives of Neurology*. 1990;47(5):586-594. doi:10.1001/archneur.1990.00530050110021.

Halperin JJ1, Little BW, Coyle PK, Dattwyler RJ. Lyme disease: cause of a treatable peripheral neuropathy. Neurology. 1987 Nov;37(11):1700-6.

Halperin JJ, Luft BJ, Anand AK, et al. Lyme neuroborreliosis: Central nervous system manifestations. *Neurology*. 1989;39(6):753-753. doi:10.1212/wnl.39.6.753.

Hammers-Berggren S, Grondahl A, Karlsson M, von Arbin M, Carlsson A, Stiernstedt G. Screening for neuroborreliosis in patients with stroke. *Stroke*. 1993;24(9):1393-1396. doi:10.1161/01.str.24.9.1393. [PubMed]

Hashimoto Y, Takahashi H, Matsuo S, Hirai K, Takemori N, Nakao M, Miyamoto K, Iizuka H. Polymerase chain reaction of Borrelia burgdorferi flagellin gene in Shulman syndrome. *Dermatology*. 1996;192(2):136-9. https://www.ncbi.nlm.nih.gov/pubmed/8829496

Hänny PE, Häuselmann HJ. [Lyme disease from the neurologist's viewpoint] [in German]. *Schweizerische medizinische Wochenschrift*. 1987;117(24):901-15. https://www.ncbi.nlm.nih.gov/pubmed/3616582. Accessed February 26, 2017. [PubMed]

Hansen K, Cruz M, Link H. Oligoclonal Borrelia burgdorjeri-specific IgG antibodies in Cerebrospinal fluid in Lyme Neuroborreliosis. *Journal of Infectious Diseases*. 1990;161(6):1194-1202. doi:10.1093/infdis/161.6.1194.

Harvey WT, Salvato P. "Lyme disease": Ancient engine of an unrecognized borreliosis pandemic? *Medical Hypotheses*. 2003;60(5):742-759. doi:10.1016/s0306-9877(03)00060-4.

Häupl T, Hahn G, Rittig M, et al. Persistence of Borrelia burgdorferi in ligamentous tissue from a patient with chronic Lyme borreliosis. *Arthritis and rheumatism*. 1993;36(11):1621-6. https://www.ncbi.nlm.nih.gov/pubmed/8240439. Accessed February 19, 2017.

Health and Consumers Directorate-General. Lyme's disease, European Commission Report, (2008). http://ec.europa.eu/health/ph_information/dissemination/echi/docs/lyme_en.pdf. Accessed February 16, 2017.

Heinrich A, Khaw AV, Ahrens N, Kirsch M, Dressel A. Cerebral Vasculitis as the only manifestation of *Borrelia burgdorferi* infection in a 17-Year-Old patient with Basal Ganglia infarction. *European Neurology*. 2003;50(2):109-112. doi:10.1159/000072510. [PubMed]

Hemmer B, Glocker F, Kaiser R, Lucking C, Deuschl G. Generalised motor neuron disease as an unusual manifestation of Borrelia burgdorferi infection. J Neurol Neurosurg Psychiatry. 1997 Aug; 63(2): 257-258. https://www.ncbi.nlm.nih.gov/pmc/articles/PMC2169663/pdf/v063p00257.pdf. Accessed February 24, 2017.

Hercogová J, Tománková M, Barták P. Contributions to the treatment of dermatologic manifestations of Lyme borreliosis. *Cutis*. 1992 Jun;49(6):409-11. https://www.ncbi.nlm.nih.gov/pubmed/1628507

Hercogová J, Vanousova D. Syphilis and borreliosis during pregnancy. *Dermatologic Therapy*. 2008;21(3):205-209. doi:10.1111/j.1529-8019.2008.00192.x.

Hercogová J, Brzonova I. Lyme disease in central Europe. *Curr Opin Infect Dis.* 2001;14(2):133-7. Review. https://www.ncbi.nlm.nih.gov/pubmed/11979122

Herman-Giddens ME. Erythema Migrans-Like lesions in the south require treatment given the current state of knowledge. *Vector-Borne and Zoonotic Diseases.* 2014;14(6):461-463. doi:10.1089/vbz.2013.1545. http://dx.doi.org/10.1089/vbz.2013.1545. Accessed January 30, 2017.

Hidri N., Barraud O., de Martino S., Garnier F., Paraf F., Martin C., Sekkal S., Laskar M., Jaulhac B.and Ploy M.-C. Lyme endocarditis. Clin. Microbiol. Infect., 18 (12) (2012), pp. E531-E532.

Hodzic E, Feng S, Holden K, Freet KJ, Barthold SW. Persistence of Borrelia burgdorferi following antibiotic treatment in mice. *Antimicrobial Agents and Chemotherapy.* 2008;52(5):1728-1736. doi:10.1128/aac.01050-07.

Hodzic E, Imai D, Feng S, Barthold SW. Resurgence of persisting Non-Cultivable Borrelia burgdorferi following antibiotic treatment in mice. *PLoS ONE.* 2014;9(1):e86907. doi:10.1371/journal.pone.0086907.

Horowitz RI, Freeman PR. Are Mycobacterium drugs effective for treatment resistant Lyme disease, tick- borne Co-Infections, and autoimmune disease? *JSM Arthritis.* 2016;1(2):1008. https://www.jscimedcentral.com/Arthritis/arthritis-1-1008.pdf. Accessed January 30, 2017.

Horowitz RI, Freeman PR. The use of Dapsone as a novel "Persister" drug in the treatment of chronic Lyme disease/post treatment Lyme disease syndrome. *Journal of Clinical and Experimental Dermatology Research.* 2016;07(03). doi:10.4172/2155-9554.1000345.

Hovius JWR, van Dam AP, Fikrig E. Tick-host-pathogen interactions in Lyme borreliosis. *Trends in Parasitology.* 2007;23(9):434-438. doi:10.1016/j.pt.2007.07.001.

Iero I, Elia M, Cosentino FII, et al. Isolated monolateral neurosensory hearing loss as a rare sign of neuroborreliosis. *Neurological Sciences.* 2004;25(1):30-33. doi:10.1007/s10072-004-0224-8. [PubMed]

Inman RD, Chiu B. Heavy metal exposure reverses genetic resistance to Chlamydia-induced arthritis. *Arthritis Research & Therapy.* 2009;11(1):R19. doi:10.1186/ar2610.

Itzhaki RF, Lathe R, Balin BJ, et al. EVIDENCE FOR AN INFECTIOUS/IMMUNE COMPONENT. *Journal of Alzheimer's Disease.* 2016;51(4):979-984. doi:10.3233/JAD-160152. http://dx.doi.org/10.3233/JAD-160152. Accessed March 1, 2017.

Johnson L, Wilcox S, Mankoff J, Stricker RB. Severity of chronic Lyme disease compared to other chronic conditions: A quality of life survey. *PeerJ.* 2014;2:e322. doi:10.7717/peerj.322.

Joseph JT, Purtill K, Wong SJ, et al. Vertical transmission of Babesia microti , United States. *Emerging Infectious Diseases.* 2012;18(8):1318-21. doi:10.3201/eid1808.110988.

Jones KL, McHugh GA, Glickstein LJ, Steere AC. Analysis of Borrelia burgdorferi genotypes in patients with Lyme arthritis: High frequency of ribosomal RNA intergenic spacer type 1 strains in antibiotic-refractory arthritis. *Arthritis Rheum.* 2009;60(7):2174-2182. doi:10.1002/art.24812.

Jovanović R, Hajrić A, Cirković A, Miković Z, Dmitrović R. [Lyme disease and pregnancy] [in Serbian]. *Glas. Srpska akademija nauka i umetnosti. Odeljenje medicinskih nauka.* 1993;43:169-72. https://www.ncbi.nlm.nih.gov/pubmed/?term=8262402. Accessed February 25, 2017.

Juchnowicz D, Rudnik I, Czernikiewicz A, Zajkowska J, Pancewicz SA. [Mental disorders in the course of lyme borreliosis and tick borne encephalitis] [in Polish]. *Przeglad epidemiologiczny.* 2002;56:37-50. https://www.ncbi.nlm.nih.gov/pubmed/12194228. Accessed March 1, 2017. [PubMed]

Kaatz M, Zelger B, Norgauer J, Ziemer M. Lymphocytic infiltration (Jessner?Kanof): Lupus erythematosus tumidus or a manifestation of borreliosis? *British Journal of Dermatology.* 2007;157(2):403-405. doi:10.1111/j.1365-2133.2007.07997.x.

Krbkova L, Stanek G. Therapy of Lyme borreliosis in children. *Infection.* 1996;24(2):170-3.

Kaciński M, Zajac A, Skowronek-Bała B, Kroczka S, Gergont A, Kubik A. CNS Lyme disease manifestation in children. *Przeglad lekarski.* 2008;64:38-40. https://www.ncbi.nlm.nih.gov/pubmed/18431910. Accessed February 27, 2017. [PubMed]

Kalish RA, Leong JM, Steere AC. Association of treatment-resistant chronic Lyme arthritis with HLA-DR4 and antibody reactivity to OspA and OspB of Borrelia burgdorferi. *Infection and Immunity.* 2003;61(7):2774-2779. http://iai.asm.org/content/61/7/2774.full.pdf. Accessed February 24, 2017.

Karadag B, Spieker LE, Schwitter J, et al. Lyme Carditis: Restitutio ad Integrum documented by cardiac...: Cardiology in review. *Cardiology in Review.* 2004;12(4):185-187. http://journals.lww.com/cardiologyinreview/Abstract/2004/07000/Lyme_Carditis_Restitutio_Ad_Integrum_Documented.2.aspx. Accessed February 13, 2017.

Karma A, Seppälä I, Mikkilä H, Kaakkola S, Viljanen M, Tarkkanen A. Diagnosis and clinical characteristics of ocular Lyme Borreliosis. *American Journal of Ophthalmology.* 1995;119(2):127-135. doi:10.1016/s0002-9394(14)73864-4.

Kathman D, Nesanelis D, Fitzgibbons C. A rare cause of Posttransfusion hemolytic anemia. *Chest.* 2013;144(4):197A-197B. doi:10.1378/chest.1700928.

Kawano Y, Shigeto H, Shiraishi Y, Ohyagi Y, Kira J. A case of Borrelia brainstem encephalitis presenting with severe dysphagia. *Rinsho Shinkeigaku.* 2010;50(4):265-267. doi:10.5692/clinicalneurol.50.265. [PubMed]

Kaya G, Berset M, Prins C, Chavaz P, Saurat JH. **Chronic** borreliosis presenting with morphea- and lichen sclerosus et atrophicus-like cutaneous lesions. a case report. *Dermatology.* 2001;202(4):373-5. DOI: 51687

Keil R, Baron R, Kaiser R, Deuschl G. [Vasculitis course of neuroborreliosis with thalamic infarct] [in German]. *Der Nervenarzt.* 1997;68(4):339-41. https://www.ncbi.nlm.nih.gov/pubmed/9273464. Accessed February 26, 2017. [PubMed]

Keymeulen B, Somers G, Naessens A, Verbruggen LA. False positive ELISA serologic test for Lyme borreliosis in patients with connective tissue diseases. *Clinical Rheumatology*. 1993;12(4):526-528. doi:10.1007/bf02231784.

Kieslich M, Fiedler A, Hernaiz Driever P, Weis R, Schwabe D, Jacobi G. Lyme borreliosis mimicking central nervous system malignancy: The diagnostic pitfall of cerebrospinal fluid cytology. *Brain and Development*. 2000;22(6):403-406. doi:10.1016/s0387-7604(00)00165-0.

Klingebiel R, Benndorf G, Schmitt M, von Moers A, Lehmann R. Large cerebral vessel occlusive disease in Lyme Neuroborreliosis. *Neuropediatrics*. 2002;33(1):37-40. doi:10.1055/s-2002-23589. [PubMed]

Koc F, Bozdemir H, Pekoz T, Aksu HS, Ozcan S, Kurdak H. Lyme disease presenting as subacute transverse myelitis. *Acta Neurol Belg*. 2009;109(4):326-329.

Kohler J, Kern U, Kasper J, Rhese-Kupper B, Thoden U. Chronic central nervous system involvement in Lyme borreliosis. *Neurology*. 1988;38(6):863-863. doi:10.1212/wnl.38.6.863.

Kohlhepp W, Kuhn W, Krüger H. Extrapyramidal features in central Lyme Borreliosis. *European Neurology*. 2008;29(3):150-155. doi:10.1159/000116399.

Kologrivova EN, Baraulina AS, Nechaeva SV, et al. [Intensity of the production of rheumatoid factor in patients with different degrees of sensitization to Borrelia garinii antigens] [in Russian]. *Zhurnal mikrobiologii, epidemiologii, i immunobiologii*. Mar-Apr 2005:80-3. https://www.ncbi.nlm.nih.gov/pubmed/15881948/. Accessed February 26, 2017.

Kostić, Tomislav ; Momčilović, Stefan ; Perišić, Zoran D. ; Apostolović, Svetlana R. ; Cvetković, Jovana ; Jovanović, Andriana ; Barać, Aleksandra ; Šalinger-Martinović, Sonja ; Tasić-Otašević, Suzana. Manifestations of Lyme carditis. Int J Cardiol. 2017 Apr 1;232:24-32. doi: 10.1016/j.ijcard.2016.12.169.

Kraemer M1, Berlit P. Systemic, secondary and infectious causes for cerebral vasculitis: clinical experience with 16 new European cases. Rheumatol Int. 2010 Sep;30(11):1471-6. doi: 10.1007/s00296-009-1172-4.

Kraiczy P. Hide and seek: How Lyme disease Spirochetes overcome complement attack. *Frontiers in Immunology*. 2016;7. doi:10.3389/fimmu.2016.00385.

Krause PJ, Hendrickson JE, Steeves TK, Fish D. Blood transfusion transmission of the tick-borne relapsing fever spirochete Borrelia miyamotoi in mice. *Transfusion*. 2014;55(3):593-597. doi:10.1111/trf.12879.

Krause PJ, Telford SR, Spielman A, et al. Concurrent Lyme disease and babesiosis. Evidence for increased severity and duration of illness. *JAMA*. 1996;275(21):1657-1660.

Krbková L, Klapačová L, Mikolášek P, Charvátová M, Červinková I, Bednářová J. Neuroborreliosis Imitating Brain Tumour in Children and Vice Versa [Největší informační zdroj pro lékaře - proLékaře.cz]. *Cesk Slov Neurol N*. 2017;77/110(5):620-623. http://www.csnn.eu/ceska-slovenskaneurologie-clanek/neuroborrelioza-imitujici-mozkovy-nador-u-deti-a-vice-versa-49684. Accessed February 23, 2017.

Krbkova L, Stanek G. Therapy of Lyme borreliosis in children. *Infection*. 1996;24(2):170-3. https://www.ncbi.nlm.nih.gov/pubmed/8740116

Krim E, Guehl D, Burbaud P, and LaguenyA. Retrobulbar optic neuritis: a complication of Lyme disease? J Neurol Neurosurg Psychiatry. 2007 Dec; 78(12): 1409-1410. doi: 10.1136/jnnp.2006.113761

Kristóf V, Bózsik B, Szirtes M, Simonyi J. Lyme borreliosis and Raynaud's syndrome. *The Lancet*. 1990;335(8695):975-976. doi:10.1016/0140-6736(90)91041-8.

Kubánek M, Šramko M, Berenová D, et al. Detection of Borrelia burgdorferi sensu lato in endomyocardial biopsy specimens in individuals with recent-onset dilated cardiomyopathy. *European Journal of Heart Failure*. 2012;14(6):588-596. doi:10.1093/eurjhf/hfs027.

Kuchynka P, Palecek T, Havranek S, Vitkova I, Nemecek E, Trckova R, Berenová D, Krsek D, Podzimkova J, Fikrle M, Danek BA, Linhart A. Recent-onset dilated cardiomyopathy associated with Borrelia burgdorferi infection. Herz. 2015 Sep;40(6):892-7. doi: 10.1007/s00059-015-4308-1.

Kugeler KJ, Griffith KS, Gould LH, et al. A review of death certificates listing Lyme disease as a cause of death in the United States. *Clinical Infectious Diseases*. 2010;52(3):364-367. doi:10.1093/cid/ciq157.

Kumar Singh S, Josef Girschick H. Molecualar survival strategies of the Lyme disease spirochete Borrelia burgdorferi. *The Lancet Infectious Diseases*. 2004;4(9):575-583. doi:10.1016/s1473-3099(04)01132-6.

Kumi-Diaka J, Harris O. Viability of Borrelia burgdorferi in storedsemen. *British Veterinary Journal*. 1995;151(2):221-224. doi:10.1016/s0007-1935(95)80015-8.

Kuntzer T, Bogousslavsky J, Miklossy J, Steck AJ, Janzer R, Regli F. Borrelia Rhombencephalomyelopathy. *Archives of Neurology*. 1991;48(8):832-836. doi:10.1001/archneur.1991.00530200072021. [PubMed]

Kurian M, Pereira VM, Vargas MI, Fluss J. Stroke-like Phenomena Revealing Multifocal Cerebral Vasculitis in Pediatric Lyme Neuroborreliosis. J Child Neurol. 2015 Aug;30(9):1226-9. doi: 10.1177/0883073814552104.

Lakos A, Solymosi N. Maternal Lyme borreliosis and pregnancy outcome. *International Journal of Infectious Diseases*. 2010;14(6):e494-e498. doi:10.1016/j.ijid.2009.07.019.

Laroche C, Lienhardt A, Boulesteix J. [Ischemic stroke caused by neuroborreliosis] [in French]. *Archives de pediatrie : organe officiel de la Societe francaise de pediatrie*. 2000;6(12):1302-5. https://www.ncbi.nlm.nih.gov/pubmed/10627902. Accessed February 26, 2017. [PubMed]

Latsch K, Tappe D, Warmuth-Metz M, Hebestreit H. Central nervous system borreliosis mimicking a pontine tumour. *Journal of Medical Microbiology*. 2006;55(11):1597-1599. doi:10.1099/jmm.0.46586-0.

Lavoie PE, Lattner BP, Duray PH, Barbour AG, Johnson HC. Culture positive seronegative transplacental Lyme borreliosis infant mortality. *Arthritis Rheum*. 1987;30(4):3(Suppl):S50.

Lebas A, Toulgoat F, Saliou G, Husson B, Tardieu M. Stroke due to Lyme Neuroborreliosis: Changes in vessel wall contrast enhancement. *Journal of Neuroimaging*. 2010;22(2):210-212. doi:10.1111/j.1552-6569.2010.00550.x. [PubMed]

Lee S, Vigliotti J, Vigliotti V, Jones W, Shearer D. Detection of Borreliae in Archived sera from patients with clinically suspect Lyme disease. *International Journal of Molecular Sciences*. 2014;15(3):4284-4298. doi:10.3390/ijms15034284.

Legatowicz-Koprowska M, Gziut A, Walczak E, Gil R, Wagner T. [Borreliosis--simultaneous Lyme carditis and psychiatric disorders--case report]. *Polski merkuriusz lekarski : organ Polskiego Towarzystwa Lekarskiego*. 2008;24(143):433-5. https://www.ncbi.nlm.nih.gov/pubmed/18634389. Accessed February 24, 2017.

Lenormand C, Jaulhac B, De Martino S, Barthel C, Lipsker D. Species of Borrelia burgdorferi complex that cause borrelial lymphocytoma in France. *Br J Dermatol*. 2009;161(1):174-6. doi: 10.1111/j.1365-2133.2009.09100.

Lesnicar G, Zerdoner D. Temporomandibular joint involvement caused by Borrelia Burgdorferi. *J Cranio-Maxillo-fac Surg Off Publ Eur Assoc Cranio-Maxillo-fac Surg*. 2007;35(8):397-400. doi:10.1016/j.jcms.2007.06.003.

Lesire V, Machet L, Toledano C, de Muret A, Maillard H, Lorette G, Vaillant L. Atypical erythema multiforme occurring at the early phase of Lyme disease? *Acta Derm Venereol*. 2000;80(3):222. https://www.ncbi.nlm.nih.gov/pubmed/10954224

Lesser RL, Kornmehl EW, Pachner AR, et al. Neuro-Ophthalmologic manifestations of Lyme disease. *Ophthalmology*. 1990;97(6):699-706. doi:10.1016/s0161-6420(90)32519-8.

Levi T, Keesing F, Oggenfuss K, Ostfeld RS. Accelerated phenology of blacklegged ticks under climate warming. *Philosophical Transactions of the Royal Society B: Biological Sciences*. 2015;370(1665):20130556-20130556. doi:10.1098/rstb.2013.0556.

Lewis K. Persister cells. *Annual Review of Microbiology*. 2010;64(1):357-372. doi:10.1146/annurev.micro.112408.134306.

Li S, Gilbert L, Harrison PA, Rounsevell MDA. Modelling the seasonality of Lyme disease risk and the potential impacts of a warming climate within the heterogeneous landscapes of Scotland. *Journal of The Royal Society Interface*. 2016;13(116). doi:10.1098/rsif.2016.0140.

Lipsker D, Hansmann Y, Limbach F, Clerc C, Tranchant C, Grunenberger F, Caro-Sampara F, Attali P, Frey M, Kubina M, Piémont Y, Sibilia J, Jaulhac B; GEBLY Study Group. Study Group for Lyme Borreliosis. Disease expression of Lyme borreliosis in northeastern France. *Eur J Clin Microbiol Infect Dis*. 2001;20(4):225-30. https://www.ncbi.nlm.nih.gov/pubmed/11399010

Louis E, Camilleri-Broët S, Crinière E, Hoang-Xuan K. Lymphomes intracrâniens du sujet immunocompétent [INTRACRANIAL IMMUNOCOMPETENT LYMPHOMAS]. *EMC - Neurologie*. 2005;2(2):204-222. doi:10.1016/j.emcn.2004.10.007.

Lyme disease. https://wonder.cdc.gov/wonder/prevguid/p0000380/p0000380.asp. Accessed January 28, 2017.

Ma Y, Sturrock A, Weis JJ. Intracellular localization of Borrelia burgdorferi within human endothelial cells. *Infect Immun*. 1991;59(2):671-678. https://www.ncbi.nlm.nih.gov/pmc/articles/PMC257809/. Accessed February 26, 2017.

MacDonald AB, Benach JL, Burgdorfer W. Stillbirth following maternal Lyme disease. *N Y State J Med*. 1987;11:615-616.

MacDonald AB, Miranda JM. Concurrent neocortical borreliosis and Alzheimer's disease. *Human Pathology*. 1987;18(7):759-761. doi:10.1016/s0046-8177(87)80252-6. [PubMed]

MacDonald AB, Miranda JM. Concurrent neocortical borreliosis and Alzheimer's disease. *Human pathology*. 1987;18(7):759-61. https://www.ncbi.nlm.nih.gov/pubmed/3297997. Accessed March 2, 2017. [PubMed]

MacDonald AB. Borrelia in the brains of patients dying with dementia. *JAMA: The Journal of the American Medical Association*. 1986;256(16):2195. doi:10.1001/jama.1986.03380160053011. [PubMed].

MacDonald AB. Concurrent Neocortical Borreliosis and Alzheimer's disease. *Annals of the New York Academy of Sciences*. 1988;539(1 Lyme Disease):468-470. doi:10.1111/j.1749-6632.1988.tb31909.x.

MacDonald AB. Gestational Lyme borreliosis. Implications for the fetus. *Rheum Dis Clin North Am*. 1989;15(4):657-677.

Macdonald AB. Human fetal borreliosis, toxemia of pregnancy, and fetal death. *Zentralblatt für Bakteriologie, Mikrobiologie und Hygiene. Series A: Medical Microbiology, Infectious Diseases, Virology, Parasitology*. 1986;263(1-2):189-200. doi:10.1016/s0176-6724(86)80122-5.

Magnusson R. *Advancing the right to health: The vital role of law*. Geneva: World Health Organization; 2017. http://apps.who.int/iris/bitstream/10665/252815/1/9789241511384-eng.pdf. Accessed February 15, 2017.

Maheshwari P, Eslick GD. Bacterial infection increases the risk of Alzheimer's disease: An evidence-based assessment. *Journal of Alzheimer's Disease*. August 2016:1-10. doi:10.3233/jad-160362.

Malane MS, Grant-Kels JM, Feder HM Jr, Luger SW. Diagnosis of Lyme disease based on dermatologic manifestations. *Ann Intern Med*. 1991;114(6):490-8. DOI: 10.7326/0003-4819-114-6-490.

Mannelli A, Bertolotti L, Gern L, Gray J. Ecology of Borrelia burgdorferi sensu lato in Europe: Transmission dynamics in multi-host systems, influence of molecular processes and effects of climate change. *FEMS Microbiology Reviews*. 2012;36(4):837-861. doi:10.1111/j.1574-6976.2011.00312.x.

Manore CA, Ostfeld RS, Agusto FB, Gaff H, LaDeau SL. Defining the risk of Zika and Chikungunya virus transmission in human population centers of the eastern United States. *PLOS Neglected Tropical Diseases*. 2017;11(1):e0005255. doi:10.1371/journal.pntd.0005255.

Maraspin V, Cimperman J, Lotric-Furlan S, Pleterski-Rigler D, Strle F. Erythema migrans in pregnancy. *Wiener klinische Wochenschrift*. 2000;111:933-40. https://www.ncbi.nlm.nih.gov/pubmed/10666804. Accessed February 13, 2017.

Maraspin V, Cimperman J, Lotric-Furlan S, Ruzić-Sabljić E, Jurca T, Picken RN, Strle F. Solitary borrelial lymphocytoma in adult patients. *Wien Klin Wochenschr*. 2002;114(13-14):515-23. https://www.ncbi.nlm.nih.gov/pubmed/12422593

Maraspin V, Nahtigal Klevišar M, Ružić-Sabljić E, Lusa L, Strle F. Borrelial Lymphocytoma in Adult Patients. *Clin Infect Dis*. 2016;63(7):914-21. doi: 10.1093/cid/ciw417

Marconi RT, Hohenberger S, Jauris-Heipke S, Schulte-Spechtel U, LaVoie CP, Rößler D, Wilske B. Genetic Analysis of Borrelia garinii OspA Serotype 4 Strains Associated with Neuroborreliosis: Evidence for Extensive Genetic Homogeneity. *J Clin Microbiol*. 1999;37(12): 3965-3970. https://www.ncbi.nlm.nih.gov/pmc/articles/PMC85856/

Markowitz LE, Steere AC, Benach JL, Slade JD, Broome CV. Lyme disease during pregnancy. *JAMA: The Journal of the American Medical Association*. 1986;255(24):3394. doi:10.1001/jama.1986.03370240064038.

Marques A, Telford SR, Turk S, et al. Xenodiagnosis to detect Borrelia burgdorferi infection: A First-in-Human study. *Clinical Infectious Diseases*. 2014;58(7):937-945. doi:10.1093/cid/cit939.

Mawanda F, Wallace R. Can infections cause Alzheimer's disease? *Epidemiologic Reviews*. 2013;35(1):161-180. doi:10.1093/epirev/mxs007.

May EF, Jabbari B. Stroke in neuroborreliosis. *Stroke*. 1990;21(8):1232-1235. doi:10.1161/01.str.21.8.1232. [PubMed]

McAlister HF. Lyme Carditis: An important cause of reversible heart block. *Annals of Internal Medicine*. 1989;110(5):339. doi:10.7326/0003-4819-110-5-339.

McManus M, Cincotta A. Effects of Borrelia on host immune system: Possible consequences for diagnostics. *Advances in Integrative Medicine*. 2015;2(2):81-89. doi:10.1016/j.aimed.2014.11.002.

Meer-Scherrer L, Chang Loa C, Adelson ME, et al. Lyme disease associated with Alzheimer's disease. *Current Microbiology*. 2006;52(4):330-332. doi:10.1007/s00284-005-0454-7. [PubMed]

Meimoun P, Sayah S, Benali T, et al. [Lyme disease presenting as infarction pain. A case report] [in French]. *Archives des maladies du coeur et des vaisseaux*. 2002;94(12):1419-22. https://www.ncbi.nlm.nih.gov/pubmed/11828929. Accessed February 13, 2017.

Melski JW, Reed KD, Mitchell PD, Barth GD. Primary and secondary erythema migrans in central Wisconsin. *Arch Dermatol*. 1993;129(6):709-16. https://www.ncbi.nlm.nih.gov/pubmed/8389536

Menni S, Pistritto G, Gelmetti C, Stanta G, Trevisan G. Eruzione a tipo pitiriasi lichenoide con perifollicoliti in corso di borreliosi di Lyme. *Eur J Pediat Dermatol*. 1994;4:77-80.

Merlo A, Weder B, Ketz E, Matter L. Locked-in state in Borrelia burgdorferi meningitis. *Journal of Neurology*. 1989;236(5):305-306. doi:10.1007/bf00314463.

Midgard R, Hofstad H. Unusual manifestations of nervous system Borrelia burgdorferi infection. *Archives of Neurology*. 1987;44(7):781-783. doi:10.1001/archneur.1987.00520190085021. [PubMed]

Mikkelse AL, Palle C. Lyme disease during pregnancy. *Acta Obstetricia et Gynecologica Scandinavica*. 1987;66(5):477-478. doi:10.3109/00016348709022058.

Mikkilä HO, Seppälä IJ, Viljanen MK, Peltomaa MP, Karma A. The expanding clinical spectrum of ocular lyme borreliosis. *Ophthalmology*. 2000;107(3):581-587.

Miklossy J, Kasas S, Janzer RC, Ardizzoni F, Van der Loos H. Further ultrastructural evidence that spirochaetes may play a role in the aetiology of Alzheimer's disease. *NeuroReport*. 1994;5(10):1201-1204. doi:10.1097/00001756-199406020-00010.

Miklossy J, Kasas S, Zurn AD, McCall S, Yu S, McGeer PL. Persisting atypical and cystic forms of Borrelia burgdorferi and local inflammation in Lyme neuroborreliosis. *Journal of Neuroinflammation*. 2008;5(1):40. doi:10.1186/1742-2094-5-40.

Miklossy J, Khalili K, Gern L, et al. Borrelia burgdorferi persists in the brain in chronic Lyme neuroborreliosis and may be associated with Alzheimer disease. *Journal of Alzheimer's Disease*. 2004;6(6):639-649. http://content.iospress.com/articles/journal-of-alzheimers-disease/jad00387. Accessed January 31, 2017. [PubMed]

Miklossy J, Kis A, Radenovic A, et al. Beta-amyloid deposition and Alzheimer's type changes induced by Borrelia spirochetes. *Neurobiology of Aging*. 2006;27(2):228-236. doi:10.1016/j.neurobiolaging.2005.01.018.

Miklossy J, Kuntzer T, Bogousslavsky J, Regli F, Janzer RC. Meningovascular form of neuroborreliosis: Similarities between neuropathological findings in a case of Lyme disease and those occurring in tertiary neurosyphilis. *Acta Neuropathologica*. 1990;80(5):568-572. doi:10.1007/bf00294622. [PubMed]

Miklossy J. Alzheimer's disease - a neurospirochetosis. Analysis of the evidence following Koch's and hill's criteria. *Journal of Neuroinflammation.* 2011;8(1):90. doi:10.1186/1742-2094-8-90. [PubMed]

Miklossy J. Alzheimer's disease--a spirochetosis? *Neuroreport.* 1993;4(7):841-8. https://www.ncbi.nlm.nih.gov/pubmed/8369471. Accessed January 31, 2017. [PubMed]

Miklossy J. Bacterial Amyloid and DNA are important constituents of senile plaques: Further evidence of the Spirochetal and Biofilm nature of senile plaques. *Journal of Alzheimer's Disease.* 2016;53(4):1459-1473. doi:10.3233/jad-160451.

Miklossy J. Biology and neuropathology of dementia in syphilis and Lyme disease. Handb Clin Neurol. 2008;89:825-44. [PubMed]

Miklossy J. Chronic inflammation and amyloidogenesis in Alzheimer's disease -- role of Spirochetes. *Journal of Alzheimer's disease : JAD.* 2008;13(4):381-91. https://www.ncbi.nlm.nih.gov/pubmed/18487847. Accessed March 1, 2017.

Miklossy J. Emerging roles of pathogens in Alzheimer disease. *Expert Reviews in Molecular Medicine.* 2011;13. doi:10.1017/s1462399411002006.

Miklossy J. Historic evidence to support a causal relationship between spirochetal infections and Alzheimer's disease. *Frontiers in Aging Neuroscience.* 2015;7:46. doi:10.3389/fnagi.2015.00046.

Miklossy J. The spirochetal etiology of Alzheimer's disease: A putative therapeutic approach. In: Giacobini E, Becker R, eds. *Proceedings of the third international Springfield Alzheimer symposium. Part I.* Birkhauser Boston Inc; 1994:41-48.

Molin S, Ruzicka T, Prinz JC. Borreliosis mimicking lupus-like syndrome during infliximab treatment. *Clinical and Experimental Dermatology.* 2010;35(6):631-633. doi:10.1111/j.1365-2230.2010.03787.x.

Moncó JCG, Wheeler CM, Benach JL, et al. Reactivity of neuroborreliosis patients (Lyme disease) to cardiolipin and gangliosides. *Journal of the Neurological Sciences.* 1993;117(1-2):206-214. doi:10.1016/0022-510x(93)90175-x.

Moritz ED, Winton CS, Tonnetti L, et al. Screening for Babesia microti in the U.S. Blood supply. *New England Journal of Medicine.* 2016;375(23):2236-2245. doi:10.1056/nejmoa1600897.

Morrison C, Seifter A, Aucott JN. Unusual presentation of Lyme disease: Horner syndrome with negative Serology. *The Journal of the American Board of Family Medicine.* 2009;22(2):219-222. doi:10.3122/jabfm.2009.02.080130.

Muehlenbachs A, Bollweg BC, Schulz TJ, et al. Cardiac Tropism of Borrelia burgdorferi. *The American Journal of Pathology.* 2016;186(5):1195-1205. doi:10.1016/j.ajpath.2015.12.027.

Munger KL, Zhang SM, O'Reilly E, et al. Vitamin D intake and incidence of multiple sclerosis. *Neurology.* 2004;62(1):60-65. doi:10.1212/01.wnl.0000101723.79681.38.

Murray R, Morawetz R, Kepes J, El Gammal T, LeDoux M. Lyme Neuroborreliosis manifesting as an Intracranial mass lesion. *Neurosurgery.* 1992;30(5):769-773. doi:10.1227/00006123-199205000-00021.

Müllegger RR, Means TK, Shin JJ, Lee M, Jones KL, Glickstein LJ, Luster AD, Steere AC. Chemokine signatures in the skin disorders of Lyme borreliosis in Europe: predominance of CXCL9 and CXCL10 in erythema migrans and acrodermatitis and CXCL13 in lymphocytoma. *Infect Immun*. 2007;75(9):4621-8. DOI: 10.1128/IAI.00263-07

Muslmani M, Gilson M, Sudre A, Juvin R, Gaudin P. [Lyme disease with hepatitis and corticosteroids: a case report]. *Rev Med Interne*. 2012;33(6):339-342. doi:10.1016/j.revmed.2012.01.016.

Mylonas I. Borreliosis during pregnancy: A risk for the unborn child? *Vector-Borne and Zoonotic Diseases*. 2011;11(7):891-898. doi:10.1089/vbz.2010.0102.

Nadal D, Hunziker UA, Bucher HU, Hitzig WH, Duc G. Infants born to mothers with antibodies against Borrelia burgdorferi at delivery. *European Journal of Pediatrics*. 1989;148(5):426-427. doi:10.1007/bf00595903.

Nadelman RB, Nowakowski J, Forseter G, et al. The clinical spectrum of early lyme borreliosis in patients with culture-confirmed erythema migrans. *The American Journal of Medicine*. 1996;100(5):502-508. doi:10.1016/s0002-9343(95)99915-9. [PubMed]

Nafeev AA, Klimova LV. [Clinical manifestations of neuroborreliosis in the Volga region]. *Ter Arkh*. 2010;82(11):68-70. https://www.ncbi.nlm.nih.gov/pubmed/21381354

Neumärker KJ, Dudeck U, Plaza P. [Borrelia encephalitis and catatonia in adolescence] [in German]. *Der Nervenarzt*. 1989;60(2):115-9. https://www.ncbi.nlm.nih.gov/pubmed/2716930. Accessed February 27, 2017. [PubMed]

Nguyen H, Le C, Nguyen H. Acute lyme infection presenting with amyopathic dermatomyositis and rapidly fatal interstitial pulmonary fibrosis: a case report. *J Med Case Reports*. 2010;4(1). doi:10.1186/1752-1947-4-187.

Nicolson GL, Haier J. Role of chronic bacterial and viral infections in neurodegenerative, neurobehavioural, psychiatric, autoimmune and fatiguing illnesses: Part 2. *British Journal of Medical Practitioners*. 2010;3(1):301. http://www.bjmp.org/files/2010-3-1/bjmp-2010-3-1-301.pdf. Accessed February 26, 2017.

Oksi J, Kalimo H, Marttila RJ, et al. Inflammatory brain changes in Lyme borreliosis. A report on three patients and review of literature. *Brain : a journal of neurology*. 1996;119:2143-54. https://www.ncbi.nlm.nih.gov/pubmed/9010017. Accessed February 19, 2017. [PubMed]

Oksi J, Viljanen MK, Kalimo H, et al. Fatal encephalitis caused by concomitant infection with tick-borne encephalitis virus and Borrelia burgdorferi. *Clinical Infectious Diseases*. 1993;16(3):392-396. doi:10.1093/clind/16.3.392. [PubMed]

Olivares J-P, Pellas F, Ceccaldi M, et al. Lyme disease presenting as isolated acute urinary retention caused by transverse myelitis: An electrophysiological and urodynamical study. *Archives of Physical Medicine and Rehabilitation*. 1995;76(12):1171-1172. doi:10.1016/s0003-9993(95)80128-6.

Olson JC, Esterly NB. Urticarial vasculitis and Lyme disease. *J Am Acad Dermatol*. 1990;22(6 Pt 1):1114-6. https://www.ncbi.nlm.nih.gov/pubmed/2370339

Olsson JE, Zbornikova V. Neuroborreliosis simulating a progressive stroke. *Acta neurologica Scandinavica*. 1990;81(5):471-4. https://www.ncbi.nlm.nih.gov/pubmed/2375251. Accessed February 26, 2017. [PubMed]

Omasits M, Seiser A, Brainin M. [Recurrent and relapsing course of borreliosis of the nervous system] [in German]. *Wiener klinische Wochenschrift*. 1990;102(1):4-12. https://www.ncbi.nlm.nih.gov/pubmed/2408240. Accessed February 27, 2017. [PubMed]

Önk G, Acun C, Kalayci M, Çağavi F, Açikgöz B, Tanriverdi HA. Gestational lyme disease as a rare cause of congenital hydrocephalus. *J Turkish German Gynecol Assoc*. 2005;6(2):156-157. http://cms.galenos.com.tr/FileIssue/27/1038/article/JTGGA-156-157.pdf. Accessed February 25, 2017.

Oschmann P, Dorndorf W, Hornig C, Schäfer C, Wellensiek HJ, Pflughaupt KW. Stages and syndromes of neuroborreliosis. *Journal of Neurology*. 1998;245(5):262-272. doi:10.1007/s004150050216. . [PubMed]

Ostfeld RS, Brunner JL. Climate change and Ixodes tick-borne diseases of humans. *Philosophical Transactions of the Royal Society B: Biological Sciences*. 2015;370(1665):20140051-20140051. doi:10.1098/rstb.2014.0051.

Ozkan S, Atabey N, Fetil E, Erkizan V, Günes AT. Evidence for Borrelia burgdorferi in morphea and lichen sclerosus. *Int J Dermatol*. 2000;39(4):278-83.
https://www.ncbi.nlm.nih.gov/pubmed/10809977

Pachner AR. Spirochetal diseases of the CNS. *Neurol Clin*. 1986;4(1):207-222.

Pachner AR, Duray P, Steere AC. Central nervous system manifestations of Lyme disease. *Archives of Neurology*. 1989;46(7):790-795. doi:10.1001/archneur.1989.00520430086023. [PubMed]

Pachner AR, Steere AC. The triad of neurologic manifestations of Lyme disease: Meningitis, cranial neuritis, and radiculoneuritis. *Neurology*. 1985;35(1):47-47. doi:10.1212/wnl.35.1.47.

Pachner AR. Borrelia burgdorferi in the nervous system: The new "great Imitator." *Annals of the New York Academy of Sciences*. 1988;539(1 Lyme Disease):56-64. doi:10.1111/j.1749-6632.1988.tb31838.x.

Pal GS, Baker JT, Humphrey PR. Lyme disease presenting as recurrent acute meningitis. *British Medical Journal*. 1987;295(6594). https://www.ncbi.nlm.nih.gov/pmc/articles/PMC1247218/pdf/bmjcred00032-0025a.pdf. Accessed February 24, 2017.

Pañczuk A, Tokarska-Rodak M, Kozioł-Montewka M, Plewik D. The incidence of Borrelia burgdorferi, Anaplasma phagocytophilum and Babesia microti coinfections among foresters and farmers in eastern Poland. *J Vector Borne Dis*. 2016;53(4):348-354.

Pausa M, Pellis V, Cinco M, et al. Serum-resistant strains of Borrelia burgdorferi evade complement-mediated killing by expressing a CD59-Like complement inhibitory molecule. *The Journal of Immunology*. 2003;170(6):3214-3222. doi:10.4049/jimmunol.170.6.3214.

Pennekamp A, Jaques M. [Chronic neuroborreliosis with gait ataxia and cognitive disorders] [in German]. *Praxis*. 1997;86(20):867-9. https://www.ncbi.nlm.nih.gov/pubmed/9312817. Accessed February 27, 2017. [PubMed]

Perronne C. Lyme and associated tick-borne diseases: Global challenges in the context of a public health threat. *Frontiers in Cellular and Infection Microbiology*. 2014;4. doi:10.3389/fcimb.2014.00074.

Pfefferkorn T, Feddersen B, Schulte-Altedorneburg G, Linn J, Pfister H-W. Tick-borne encephalitis with polyradiculitis documented by MRI. *Neurology*. 2007;68(15):1232-1233. doi:10.1212/01.wnl.0000259065.58968.10. [PubMed]

Picken RN, Strle F, Ruzic-Sabljic E, et al. Molecular Subtyping of Borrelia burgdorferi sensu lato isolates from Five patients with solitary Lymphocytoma. *Journal of Investigative Dermatology*. 1997;108(1):92-97. doi:10.1111/1523-1747.ep12285646.

Pitassi LHU, de Paiva Diniz PPV, Scorpio DG, et al. Bartonella spp. Bacteremia in blood donors from Campinas, brazil. *PLOS Neglected Tropical Diseases*. 2015;9(1):e0003467. doi:10.1371/journal.pntd.0003467.

Ponz E, Graus F, Alvarez R, Sarmiento X, Vidal J, Grau JM. [Meningoencephalomyelitis caused by Borrelia burgdorferi: A case without epidemiologic history or chronic migratory erythema] [in Spanish]. *Medicina clinica*. 1989;93(6):218-20. https://www.ncbi.nlm.nih.gov/pubmed/2601480. Accessed February 27, 2017. [PubMed]

Preac-Mursic V, Weber K, Pfister H, et al. Survival of Borrelia burgdorferi in antibiotically treated patients with Lyme borreliosis. *Infection*. 1989;17(6):355-9. https://www.ncbi.nlm.nih.gov/pubmed/2613324. Accessed February 19, 2017.

Qiu W-G, Schutzer SE, Bruno JF, et al. Genetic exchange and plasmid transfers in Borrelia burgdorferi sensu stricto revealed by three-way genome comparisons and multilocus sequence typing. *Proceedings of the National Academy of Sciences of the United States of America*. 2004;101(39):14150-14155. doi:10.1073/pnas.0402745101. http://www.pnas.org/content/101/39/14150.long. Accessed February 18, 2017.

Radolf JD, Bourell KW, Akins DR, Brusca JS, Norgard MV. Analysis of Borrelia burgdorferi membrane architecture by freeze-fracture electron microscopy. *Journal of Bacteriology*. 1994;176(1):21-31. doi:10.1128/jb.176.1.21-31.1994.

Reik L, Burgdorfer W, Donaldson JO. Neurologic abnormalities in lyme disease without erythema chronicum migrans. *The American Journal of Medicine*. 1986;81(1):73-78. doi:10.1016/0002-9343(86)90185-3. [PubMed]

Reik L. Stroke due to Lyme disease. *Neurology*. 1993;43(12):2705-2705. doi:10.1212/wnl.43.12.2705. [PubMed]

Renaud I, Cachin C, Gerster J-C. Good outcomes of Lyme arthritis in 24 patients in an endemic area of Switzerland. *Jt Bone Spine Rev Rhum*. 2004;71(1):39-43. doi:10.1016/S1297-319X(03)00160-X.

Rey V, Du Pasquier R, Muehl A, Péter O, Michel P. [Multiple ischemic strokes due to Borrelia garinii meningovasculitis] [in French]. *Revue Neurologique*. 2010;166(11):931-934. doi:10.1016/j.neurol.2010.03.010. [PubMed]

Riviere GR, Riviere KH, Smith KS. Molecular and immunological evidence of oral Treponema in the human brain and their association with Alzheimer's disease. *Oral Microbiology and Immunology*. 2002;17(2):113-118. doi:10.1046/j.0902-0055.2001.00100.x.

Rogers HJ. Short notes and clinical cases: the question of silver cells as proof of the spirochaetal theory of disseminated sclerosis. *Journal of Neurology, Neurosurgery & Psychiatry*. 1932;s1-13(49):50-51. doi:10.1136/jnnp.s1-13.49.50.

Romi F, Kråkenes J, Aarli JA, Tysnes OB. Neuroborreliosis with Vasculitis causing stroke-like manifestations. *European Neurology*. 2004;51(1):49-50. doi:10.1159/000075090. [PubMed]

Rostoff P, Konduracka E, Massri E, et al. [Lyme carditis presenting as acute coronary syndrome: A case report] [in Polish]. *Kardiologia polska*. 2008;66(4):420-5. https://www.ncbi.nlm.nih.gov/pubmed/18473271. Accessed February 13, 2017.

Roush JK, Manley PA, Dueland RT. Rheumatoid arthritis subsequent to Borrelia burgdorferi infection in two dogs. *J Am Vet Med Assoc*. 1980;195(7):951-3.

Rudenko N, Golovchenko M, Grubhoffer L, Oliver JH. Updates on Borrelia burgdorferi sensu lato complex with respect to public health. *Ticks and Tick-borne Diseases*. 2011;2(3):123-128. doi:10.1016/j.ttbdis.2011.04.002.

Rudenko N, Golovchenko M, Mokracek A, et al. Detection of Borrelia bissettii in cardiac valve tissue of a patient with Endocarditis and Aortic valve Stenosis in the Czech Republic. *Journal of Clinical Microbiology*. 2008;46(10):3540-3543. doi:10.1128/jcm.01032-08.

Rudenko N, Golovchenko M, Vancova M, Clark K, Grubhoffer L, Oliver JH. Isolation of live Borrelia burgdorferi sensu lato spirochaetes from patients with undefined disorders and symptoms not typical for Lyme borreliosis. *Clinical Microbiology and Infection*. 2016;22(3):267.e9-267.e15. doi:10.1016/j.cmi.2015.11.009.

Ruitenberg A, Fight CJ, van den Bent MJ, Taal W. Klinisch denken en beslissen in de praktijk. Een oudere man met prostaatcarcinoom en een pijnloze parese aan de benen [Clinical thinking and decision making in practice. An elderly man with prostate cancer and a painless paresis in the legs].

Nederlands tijdschrift voor geneeskunde. 2008;149(32):1785-1790. https://www.ntvg.nl/artikelen/klinisch-denken-en-beslissen-de-praktijk-een-oudere-man-met-prostaatcarcinoom-en-een/volledig. Accessed February 24, 2017.

Ryberg B. Bannwarth's syndrome (lymphocytic meningoradiculitis) in Sweden. *Yale Journal of Biology and Medicine*. 1984;57(4). https://www.ncbi.nlm.nih.gov/pmc/articles/PMC2590032/. Accessed February 24, 2017.

Sapi E, Balasubramanian K, Poruri A, et al. Evidence of in vivo existence of Borrelia biofilm in borrelial lymphocytomas. *European Journal of Microbiology and Immunology*. 2016;6(1):9-24. doi:10.1556/1886.2015.00049.

Sapi E, Bastian SL, Mpoy CM, et al. Characterization of Biofilm formation by Borrelia burgdorferi in vitro. *PLoS ONE*. 2012;7(10):e48277. doi:10.1371/journal.pone.0048277.

Sapi E, MacDonald A. Biofilms of Borrelia burgdoferi in chronic cutaneous borreliosis. *Am J Clin Pathol*. 2008;129:988-989.

Sauer A, Hansmann Y, Jaulhac B, Bourcier T, Speeg-SchatzClaude. Five cases of Paralytic Strabismus as a rare feature of Lyme disease. *Clinical Infectious Diseases*. 2009;48(6):756-759. doi:10.1086/597041.

Saulsbury FT. Lyme arthritis in 20 children residing in a non-endemic area. *Clinical Pediatrics*. 2005;44(5):419-421. doi:10.1177/000992280504400506.

Sauvant G, Bossart W, Kurrer M, Follath F. [Diagnosis and course of myocarditis: A survey in the medical clinics of Zurich university hospital 1980 to 1998] [in German]. *Schweizerische medizinische Wochenschrift*. 2000;130(36):1265-71. https://www.ncbi.nlm.nih.gov/pubmed/11028270. Accessed February 13, 2017.

Schaeffer S, Le Doze F, De la Sayette V, Bertran F, Viader F. [Dementia in Lyme disease] [in France]. *Presse medicale (Paris, France : 1983)*. 1994;23(18). https://www.ncbi.nlm.nih.gov/pubmed/7937612. Accessed March 1, 2017. [PubMed]

Schefte DF, Nordentoft T. Intestinal Pseudoobstruction caused by chronic Lyme Neuroborreliosis. A case report. *Journal of Neurogastroenterology and Motility*. 2015;21(3):440-442. doi:10.5056/jnm14118.

Schempp C, Bocklage H, Lange R, Kölmel HW, Orfanos CE, Gollnick H. Further evidence for Borrelia burgdorferi infection in morphea and lichen sclerosus et atrophicus confirmed by DNA amplification. *J Invest Dermatol*. 1993;100(5):717-20. https://www.ncbi.nlm.nih.gov/pubmed/?term=8491994

Schlesinger PA, Duray PH, Burke BA, Steere AC, Stillman MT. Maternal-fetal transmission of the Lyme disease Spirochete, Borrelia burgdorferi. *Annals of Internal Medicine*. 1985;103(1):67. doi:10.7326/0003-4819-103-1-67.

Schmid GP. Epidemiology and clinical similarities of human spirochetal diseases. *Rev Infect Dis*. 1989;11Suppl 6:S1460-9. https://www.ncbi.nlm.nih.gov/pubmed/2682958

Schmiedel J, Gahn G, von Kummer R, Reichmann H. Cerebral Vasculitis with multiple Infarcts caused by Lyme disease. *Cerebrovascular Diseases*. 2003;17(1):79-80. doi:10.1159/000073904. [PubMed]

Schmitt AB, Küker W, Nacimiento W. [Neuroborreliosis with extensive cerebral vasculitis and multiple cerebral infarcts] [in German]. *Der Nervenarzt*. 1999;70(2):167-71.
https://www.ncbi.nlm.nih.gov/pubmed/10098153. Accessed February 26, 2017. [PubMed]

Schnarr S, Putschky N, Jendro MC, et al. Chlamydia and Borrelia DNA in synovial fluid of patients with early undifferentiated oligoarthritis: results of a prospective study. *Arthritis Rheum*. 2001;44(11):2679-2685.

Schollkopf C, Melbye M, Munksgaard L, et al. Borrelia infection and risk of non-hodgkin lymphoma. *Blood*. 2008;111(12):5524-5529. doi:10.1182/blood-2007-08-109611.

Schutzer SE, Janniger CK, Schwartz RA. Lyme disease during pregnancy. *Cutis*. 1991;47(4):267-8.
https://www.ncbi.nlm.nih.gov/pubmed/2070648. Accessed February 25, 2017.

Schwarzenbach R, Djawari D. [Pseudopelade Brocq--possible sequela of stage III Borrelia infection?] [in German]. *Der Hautarzt; Zeitschrift fur Dermatologie, Venerologie, und verwandte Gebiete*. 1999;49(11):835-7. https://www.ncbi.nlm.nih.gov/pubmed/9879482. Accessed February 13, 2017.

Schwarzova K, Kozub P, Szep Z, Golovchenko M, Rudenko N. Detection of Borrelia burgdorferi sensu stricto and Borrelia garinii DNAs in patient with Hyperkeratosis lenticularis perstans (Flegel disease). *Folia Microbiologica*. 2016;61(5):359-363. doi:10.1007/s12223-016-0444-0.

Sethi S, Alcid D, Kesarwala H, Tolan RW. Probable congenital Babesiosis in infant, new jersey, USA. *Emerging Infectious Diseases*. 2009;15(5):788-791. doi:10.3201/eid1505.070808.

Shadick NA, Phillips CB, Logigian EL, et al. The long-term clinical outcomes of Lyme disease. A population-based retrospective cohort study. *Annals of internal medicine*. 1994;121(8):560-7.
https://www.ncbi.nlm.nih.gov/pubmed/8085687. Accessed February 27, 2017. [PubMed]

Shapiro ED. Repeat or persistent Lyme disease: Persistence, recrudescence or reinfection with Borrelia Burgdorferi? *F1000Prime Reports*. 2015;7. doi:10.12703/p7-11.

Sharma B, Brown AV, Matluck NE, Hu LT, Lewis K. Borrelia burgdorferi, the causative agent of Lyme disease, forms drug-tolerant Persister cells. *Antimicrobial Agents and Chemotherapy*. 2015;59(8):4616-4624. doi:10.1128/aac.00864-15.

Sharma B, Brown AV, Matluck NE, Hu LT, Lewis K. Borrelia burgdorferi, the causative agent of Lyme disease, forms drug-tolerant Persister cells. *Antimicrobial Agents and Chemotherapy*. 2015;59(8):4616-4624. doi:10.1128/aac.00864-15.

Signs and symptoms of Lyme disease. In: McFadzean N. *The beginner's guide to Lyme disease: Diagnosis and treatment made simple*. San Diego, CA, United States: BioMed Publishing Group; October 15, 2012:67-78chap 9. ISBN-13: 9780988243712.

Silver HM. Lyme disease during pregnancy. *Infectious Disease Clinics of North America*. 1997;11(1):93-97. doi:10.1016/s0891-5520(05)70343-3.

Silver RM, Yang L, Daynes RA, Branch WD, Salafia CM, Weis JJ. Fetal outcome in Murine Lyme disease. *Infection and Immunity*. 1995;63(1):66-72. http://iai.asm.org/content/63/1/66.full.pdf. Accessed February 13, 2017.

Simecka JW, Ross SE, Cassell GH, Davis JK. Interactions of Mycoplasmas with B cells: Antibody production and nonspecific effects. *Clinical Infectious Diseases*. 1993;17(Supplement 1):S176-S182. doi:10.1093/clinids/17.supplement_1.s176.

Singh SK, Girschick HJ. Molecualar survival strategies of the Lyme disease spirochete Borrelia burgdorferi. *The Lancet Infectious Diseases*. 2004;4(9):575-583. doi:10.1016/s1473-3099(04)01132-6.

Smith AJ, Oertle J, Prato D. Chronic Lyme disease: Persistent clinical symptoms related to immune evasion, antibiotic resistance and various defense mechanisms of *Borrelia burgdorferi*. *Open Journal of Medical Microbiology*. 2014;04(04):252-260. doi:10.4236/ojmm.2014.44029. http://file.scirp.org/pdf/OJMM_2014123116044156.pdf. Accessed January 30, 2017.

Spach DH, Shimada JK, Paauw DS. Localized alopecia at the site of erythema migrans. *Journal of the American Academy of Dermatology*. 1992;27(6):1023-1024. doi:10.1016/s0190-9622(08)80275-7.

Sparsa L, Blanc F, Lauer V, Cretin B, Marescaux C, Wolff V. [Recurrent ischemic strokes revealing Lyme meningovascularitis] [in French]. *Revue Neurologique*. 2009;165(3):273-277. doi:10.1016/j.neurol.2008.06.010.. [PubMed]

Spencer JC, Eschweiler C, Butler AW. Report #1 on Lyme disease, a series. Houston, TX: The Endowment for Medical Research; 2006. http://www.endowmentmed.org/pdf/updatelyme.pdf. Accessed February 24, 2017.

Sriram S, Stratton CW, YaoSong-Yi, et al. Chlamydia pneumoniae infection of the central nervous system in multiple sclerosis. *Annals of Neurology*. 1999;46(1):6-14. doi:10.1002/1531-8249(199907)46:1<6::aid-ana4>3.3.co;2-d.

Standards Committee, Institute of Medicine, Board on Health Care Services. *Clinical practice guidelines we can trust*. Graham R, Mancher M, Miller Wolman D, Greenfield S, Steinberg E, eds. Washington, DC: National Academies Press; June 16, 2011.

Stanek G, Klein J, Bittner R, Glogar D. Borrelia burgdorferi as an etiologic agent in chronic heart failure? *Scandinavian journal of infectious diseases. Supplementum*. 1991;77:85-7. https://www.ncbi.nlm.nih.gov/pubmed/1947816. Accessed February 13, 2017.

Steere A, Malawista S, Snydman, Shope R, Andiman W, Steele F. Lyme arthritis: An epidemic of oligoarticular arthritis in children and adults in three Connecticut communities. *Arthritis and rheumatism*. 1977;20(1):7-17. https://www.ncbi.nlm.nih.gov/pubmed/836338. Accessed February 15, 2017.

Steere AC, Dwyer E, Winchester R. Association of chronic Lyme arthritis with HLA-DR4 and HLA-DR2 Alleles. *New England Journal of Medicine*. 1990;323(4):219-223. doi:10.1056/nejm199007263230402.

Steere AC, Klitz W, Drouin EE, et al. Antibiotic-refractory Lyme arthritis is associated with HLA-DR molecules that bind aBorrelia burgdorferipeptide. *The Journal of Experimental Medicine*. 2006;203(4):961-971. doi:10.1084/jem.20052471.

Steere AC. The early clinical manifestations of Lyme disease. *Annals of Internal Medicine*. 1983;99(1):76. doi:10.7326/0003-4819-99-1-76.

Steiner G. Acute plaques in multiple sclerosis, their Pathogenetic significance and the role of Spirochetes as Etiological factor. *Journal of Neuropathology & Experimental Neurology*. 1952;11(4):343-372. doi:10.1097/00005072-195210000-00001.

Steiner G. Morphology of Spirochaeta myelophthora in multiple sclerosis. *Journal of neuropathology and experimental neurology*. 1954;13(1):221-9. https://www.ncbi.nlm.nih.gov/pubmed/13118387. Accessed February 26, 2017.

Straubinger R, Summers B, Chang Y, Appel M. Persistence of Borrelia burgdorferi in experimentally infected dogs after antibiotic treatment. *Journal of clinical microbiology*. 1997;35(1):111-6. https://www.ncbi.nlm.nih.gov/pubmed/8968890. Accessed February 19, 2017.

Stricker RB, Johnson L. Let's tackle the testing. *British Medical Journal*. 2007;335(7628):1008. doi:10.1136/bmj.39394.676227.BE. http://dx.doi.org/10.1136/bmj.39394.676227.BE. Accessed February 18, 2017.

Stricker RB, Moore DH, Winger EE. Clinical and immunologic evidence for transmission of Lyme disease through intimate human contact. *J Invest Med*. 2004;52(S151).

Strle F, Maraspin V, Pleterski-Rigler D, Lotric-Furlan S, Ruzić-Sabljić E, Jurca T, Cimperman J. Treatment of borrelial lymphocytoma. Infection. 1996;24(1):80-4.
https://www.ncbi.nlm.nih.gov/pubmed/8852477

Strobino B, Abid S, Gewitz M. Maternal Lyme disease and congenital heart disease: A case-control study in an endemic area. *American Journal of Obstetrics and Gynecology*. 1999;180(3):711-716. doi:10.1016/s0002-9378(99)70277-2.

Strobino BA, Williams CL, Abid S, Ghalson R, Spierling P. Lyme disease and pregnancy outcome: A prospective s of two thousand prenatal patients. *American Journal of Obstetrics and Gynecology*. 1993;169(2):367-374. doi:10.1016/0002-9378(93)90088-z.

Sultan P, Green C, Riley E, Carvalho B. Spinal anaesthesia for caesarean delivery in a parturient with babesiosis and Lyme disease. *Anaesthesia*. 2012;67(2):180-183. doi:10.1111/j.1365-2044.2011.06941.x.

Summerday NM, Brown SJ, Allington DR, Rivey MP. Vitamin D and multiple sclerosis: Review of a possible association. *Journal of Pharmacy Practice*. 2011;25(1):75-84. doi:10.1177/0897190011421839.

Tager FA, Fallon BA, Keilp J, Rissenberg M, Jones CR, Liebowitz MR. A controlled study of cognitive deficits in children with chronic Lyme disease. *The Journal of Neuropsychiatry and Clinical Neurosciences*. 2001;13(4):500-507. doi:10.1176/jnp.13.4.500.

Tarasów E, Ustymowicz A, Zajkowska J, Hermanowska-Szpakowicz T. [Neuroborreliosis: CT and MRI findings in 14 cases. Preliminary communication] [in Polish]. *Neurologia i neurochirurgia polska*. 2002;35(5):803-13. https://www.ncbi.nlm.nih.gov/pubmed/11873593. Accessed March 1, 2017. . [PubMed

Thorp AM, Tonnetti L. Distribution and survival of Borrelia miyamoto iin human blood components. *Transfusion*. 2015;56(3):705-711. doi:10.1111/trf.13398.

Topakian R, Stieglbauer K, Aichner FT. Unexplained cerebral vasculitis and stroke: Keep Lyme neuroborreliosis in mind. *The Lancet Neurology*. 2007;6(9):756-757. doi:10.1016/s1474-4422(07)70203-x. [PubMed]

Topakian R, Stieglbauer K, Nussbaumer K, Aichner FT (2008) Cerebral vasculitis and stroke in Lyme neuroborreliosis. Cerebr Dis 26:455-461.

Trevisan G, Rees DH, Stinco G. Morphea Borrelia burgdorferi and localized scleroderma. Clin Dermatol. 1994;12(3):475-9. http://dx.doi.org/10.1016/0738-081X(94)90300-X

U.S. Centers for Disease Control and Prevention. Lyme disease surveillance and available data. Lyme disease. https://www.cdc.gov/lyme/stats/survfaq.html. Accessed February 15, 2017.

U.S. Centers for Disease Control and Prevention. Syphilis - CDC fact sheet. https://www.cdc.gov/std/syphilis/stdfact-syphilis.htm. Accessed February 15, 2017.

U.S. Environmental Protection Agency. Climate change indicators: Lyme disease. Climate Change Indicators. https://www.epa.gov/climate-indicators/climate-change-indicators-lyme-disease. Accessed February 18, 2017.

Uldry PA, Regli F, Bogousslavsky J. Cerebral angiopathy and recurrent strokes following Borrelia burgdorferi infection. *Journal of Neurology, Neurosurgery & Psychiatry*. 1987;50(12):1703-1704. doi:10.1136/jnnp.50.12.1703. [PMC free article] [PubMed]

United Nations Office of the Special Advisor on Africa (OSAA) and the NEPAD-OECD Africa Investment Initiative. Africa Fact Sheet Main Economic Indicators, United Nations Office of the Special Adviser on Africa, (2005).https://www.oecd.org/investment/investmentfordevelopment/47452483.pdf. Accessed February 18, 2017.

van Dop WA, Kersten M, de Wever B, Hovius JW. Seronegative Lyme neuroborreliosis in a patient using rituximab. *Case Reports*. 2013;2013(feb14 1):bcr2012007627-bcr2012007627. doi:10.1136/bcr-2012-007627.

van Holten J, Tiems J, Jongen VHWM. Neonatal Borrelia duttoni infection: A report of three cases. *Tropical Doctor*. 1997;27(2):115-116. doi:10.1177/004947559702700229.

Van Snick S, Duprez TP, Kabamba B, Van De Wyngaert FA, Sindic CJ. Acute ischaemic pontine stroke revealing lyme neuroborreliosis in a young adult. *Acta neurologica Belgica*. 2009;108(3):103-6. https://www.ncbi.nlm.nih.gov/pubmed/19115674. Accessed February 27, 2017. [PubMed]

Vasudevan B, Sagar A, Bahal A, Mohanty AP. Extragenital lichen sclerosus with aetiological link to Borrelia. MJAFI. 2011;67:370-3. doi: 10.1016/S0377-1237(11)60089-0.

Vasudevan B, Chatterjee M. Lyme Borreliosis and Skin. *Indian J Dermatol*. 2013;58(3): 167-174. doi: 10.4103/0019-5154.110822

Veenendaal-Hilbers JA, M. Perquin WV, Hoogland PH, Doornbos L. Basal meningo-vasculitis and occlusion of the basilar artery in two cases of Borrelia burgdorferi infection. *Neurology*. 1988;38(8):1317-1317. doi:10.1212/wnl.38.8.1317. [PubMed]

Verma V, Roman M, Shah D, Zaretskaya M, Yassin MH. A case of chronic progressive Lyme encephalitis as a manifestation of late Lyme neuroborreliosis. *Infectious Disease Reports*. 2014;6(4). doi:10.4081/idr.2014.5496.

Vos FI, Merkus P, van Nieuwkerk EBJ, Hensen EF. Rare cause of bilateral sudden deafness. *BMJ Case Reports*. October 2016:bcr2016216004. doi:10.1136/bcr-2016-216004.

Wackernagel A, Bergmann A, Aberer E. Acute exacerbation of systemic scleroderma in Borrelia burgdorferi infection. *Journal of the European Academy of Dermatology and Venereology*. 2005;19(1):93-96. doi:10.1111/j.1468-3083.2004.01074.x.

Waisbren BA, Cashman N, Schell RF, Johnson R. Borrelia burgdorferi antibodies and amyotrophic lateral sclerosis. *The Lancet*. 1987;330(8554):332-333. doi:10.1016/s0140-6736(87)90917-2.

Walsh CA, Mayer EW, Baxi LV. Lyme disease in pregnancy: Case report and review of the literature. *Obstetrical & Gynecological Survey*. 2007;62(1):41-50. doi:10.1097/01.ogx.0000251024.43400.9a.

Walther EU, Seelos K, Bise K, Mayer M, Straube A. Lyme Neuroborreliosis mimicking primary CNS lymphoma. *European Neurology*. 2004;51(1):43-45. doi:10.1159/000075086.

Waniek C, Prohovnik I, Kaufman MA, Dwork AJ. Rapidly progressive frontal-type dementia associated with Lyme disease. *The Journal of Neuropsychiatry and Clinical Neurosciences*. 1995;7(3):345-347. doi:10.1176/jnp.7.3.345. [PubMed]

Watanakunakorn C, Toliver J. Lyme arthritis with Subarticular cyst formation in Metacarpal and Metatarsal bones. *Southern Medical Journal*. 1992;85(2):187-188. doi:10.1097/00007611-199202000-00016.

Watzinger N, Fruhwald F, Schafhalter I, et al. [Coronary aneurysm in a 69-year-old patient. Transthoracic echocardiography] [in German]. *Ultraschall in der Medizin - European Journal of Ultrasound*. 1995;16(04):200-202. doi:10.1055/s-2007-1003939.

Weber K, Bratzke H-J, Neubert U, Wilske B, Duray PH. Borrelia burgdorferi in a newborn despite oral penicillin for Lyme borreliosis during pregnancy. *The Pediatric Infectious Disease Journal*. 1988;7(4):286-288. doi:10.1097/00006454-198804000-00010.

Weder B, Wiedersheim P, Matter L, Steck A, Otto F. Chronic progressive neurological involvement in Borrelia burgdorferi infection. *Journal of Neurology*. 1987;234(1):40-43. doi:10.1007/bf00314008. [PubMed]

Weigelt W, Schneider T, Lange R. Sequence homology between spirochaete flagellin and human myelin basic protein. *Immunology Today*. 1992;13(7):279-280. doi:10.1016/0167-5699(92)90012-v.

Weiss NL, Sadock VA, Sigal LH, Phillips M, Merryman PF, Abramson SB. False positive seroreactivity to Borrelia burgdorferi in systemic lupus erythematosus: The value of immunoblot analysis. *Lupus*. 1995;4(2):131-137. doi:10.1177/096120339500400209.

Wendling D, Sevrin P, Bouchaud-Chabot A, et al. Parsonage-Turner syndrome revealing Lyme borreliosis. *Jt Bone Spine Rev Rhum*. 2009;76(2):202-204. doi:10.1016/j.jbspin.2008.07.013.

Whitmire WM, Garon CF. Specific and nonspecific responses of murine B cells to membrane blebs of Borrelia burgdorferi. *Infection and Immunity*. 1993;61(4):1460-1467. http://www.ncbi.nlm.nih.gov/pmc/articles/PMC281386/.

Wienecke R1, Zöchling N, Neubert U, Schlüpen EM, Meurer M, Volkenandt M. Molecular subtyping of Borrelia burgdorferi in erythema migrans and acrodermatitis chronica atrophicans. *J Invest Dermatol*. 1994;103(1):19-22. https://www.ncbi.nlm.nih.gov/pubmed/8027576

Wilder RL, Crofford LJ. Do Infectious Agents Cause Rheumatoid Arthritis?. *Clinical Orthopaedics and Related Research*. 1991;265:36-41 http://journals.lww.com/corr/Fulltext/1991/04000/Do_Infectious_Agents_Cause_Rheumatoid_Arthritis__.5.aspx.

Williams Cl, Strobino B, Lee A, et al. Lyme disease in childhood: Clinical and epidemiologic features of ninety cases. *The Pediatric Infectious Disease Journal*. 1990;9(1):10-14. doi:10.1097/00006454-199001000-00003.

Williams CL, Strobino B, Weinstein A, Spierling P, Medici F. Maternal Lyme disease and congenital malformations: A cord blood serosurvey in endemic and control areas. *Paediatric and Perinatal Epidemiology*. 1995;9(3):320-330. doi:10.1111/j.1365-3016.1995.tb00148.x.

Wittwer B, Pelletier S, Ducrocq X, Maillard L, Mione G, Richard S. Cerebrovascular Events in Lyme Neuroborreliosis. J Stroke Cerebrovasc Dis. 2015 Jul;24(7):1671-8. doi: 10.1016/j.jstrokecerebrovasdis.2015.03.056.

Wu Q, Guan G, Liu Z, Li Y, Luo J, Yin H. RNA-Seq-based analysis of changes in Borrelia burgdorferi gene expression linked to pathogenicity. *Parasites & Vectors*. 2015;8(1):155. doi:10.1186/s13071-014-0623-2.

Wu X-B, Na R-H, Wei S-S, Zhu J-S, Peng H-J. Distribution of tick-borne diseases in china. *Parasites & Vectors*. 2013;6(1):119. doi:10.1186/1756-3305-6-119.

Yoshinari NH, de Barros PJ, Bonoldi VL, Ishikawa M, Battesti DM, Pirana S, da Fonseca AH, Schumaker TT. [Outline of Lyme borreliosis in Brazil]. *Rev Hosp Clin Fac Med Sao Paulo*. 1997;52(2):111-7. https://www.ncbi.nlm.nih.gov/pubmed/9435406

Zajkowska J1, Garkowski A, Moniuszko A, Czupryna P, Ptaszyńska-Sarosiek I, Tarasów E, Ustymowicz A, Łebkowski W, Pancewicz S. Vasculitis and stroke due to Lyme neuroborreliosis - a review. Infect Dis (Lond). 2015 Jan;47(1):1-6. doi: 10.3109/00365548.2014.961544.

Zanchi AC, Gingold AR, Theise ND, Min AD. Necrotizing Granulomatous hepatitis as an unusual manifestation of Lyme disease. *Digestive Diseases and Sciences*. 2007;52(10):2629-2632. doi:10.1007/s10620-006-9405-9.

Zhang Y, Lafontant G, Bonner FJ. Lyme neuroborreliosis mimics stroke: A case report. *Archives of Physical Medicine and Rehabilitation*. 2000;81(4):519-521. doi:10.1053/mr.2000.4431. [PubMed]

Zhang Y. Persisters, persistent infections and the Yin-Yang model. *Emerging Microbes & Infections*. 2014;3(1):e3. doi:10.1038/emi.2014.3.

Zinchuk AN, Kalyuzhna LD, Pasichna IA. Is Localized Scleroderma Caused by Borrelia burgdorferi? *Vector Borne Zoonotic Dis*. 2016;16(9):577-80. doi: 10.1089/vbz.2016.2004.

30 YEARS AND COUNTING

V International Conference on Lyme Borreliosis

PROGRAM AND ABSTRACTS

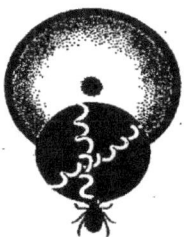

Arlington, Virginia, U.S.A.
May 30-June 2, 1992
Hyatt Regency Crystal City

63

CULTURE-CONFIRMED TREATMENT FAILURE OF CEFOTAXIME AND MINOCYCLINE IN A CASE OF LYME MENINGOENCEPHALOMYELITIS IN THE UNITED STATES.

Kenneth B. Liegner, Carl E. Rosenkilde, Grant L. Campbell*, Thomas J. Quan, and David T. Dennis, Armonk, NY, USA, Mount Kisco, NY, USA, and Centers for Disease Control, Fort Collins, CO, USA.

In 1987, a 37-year-old woman living in Westchester County, NY, developed spastic paraparesis, bilateral Babinski reflexes, and cranial nerve and bulbar dysfunction characterized by dysphagia, dysphonia, diplopia, absent gag reflex, and dysfunction of bowel and bladder control. CSF contained 19 WBC/mm^3 (86% lymphs). A test for antibodies to *Borrelia burgdorferi* (*Bb*) in serum was negative. No etiology was established despite an extensive workup. Symptoms and signs reportedly worsened gradually from 1988 to present. There was a past history of splenectomy for idiopathic thrombocytopenic purpura diagnosed in 1975. In 1989, the right frontal region and right basal ganglia were abnormal on brain MRI. In January 1990, CSF contained 6 WBC/mm^3 (93% lymphs), but no oligoclonal bands or myelin basic protein. Paired CSF and serum tests for antibodies to *Bb*, and PCR for *Bb*-specific oligonucleotides in CSF, were negative. An empiric 21-day course of cefotaxime (3 g/12 hr i.v.) was given in January, 1990 with no clear clinical benefit. Following treatment, CSF contained 9 WBC/mm^3 (93% lymphs). Four months of minocycline (200 mg/day p.o.) begun in November, 1990 also yielded no clear clinical benefit. In December, 1990 a T-cell stimulation test with *Bb* antigens was strongly positive. In December, 1991 CSF contained 6 WBC/mm^3 (89% lymphs) and elevated IgG. Paired serum and CSF samples were strongly positive for antibodies to *Bb*, with a CSF-to-serum index of 1.04. Culture of this CSF specimen in BSK-II yielded a strain of *Bb*. Culture-confirmed treatment failures have been previously reported for three Lyme neuroborreliosis cases in Europe. The present case apparently is the first of this type to be reported from the United States.

www.ingramcontent.com/pod-product-compliance
Lightning Source LLC
Chambersburg PA
CBHW082344220526
45470CB00008B/2630